IMMUNOLOGY AND IMMUNE SYSTEM DISORDERS

# IMMUNOLOGY IN CLINIC PRACTICE

# IMMUNOLOGY AND IMMUNE SYSTEM DISORDERS

**Chronic Fatigue Syndrome: Symptoms, Causes and Prevention**
*Edita Svoboda and Kristof Zelenjcik (Editors)*
2009. ISBN: 978-1-60741-493-3

**Quantitative Immunohistology: Problems and Solutions**
*Anthony S-Y Leong and, Trishe Y-M Leong*
2010. ISBN: 978-1-61668-611-6

**Autoimmune Diseases: Symptoms, Diagnosis and Treatment**
*Kyle J. Brenner (Editor)*
2010. ISBN: 978-1-61668-007-7

**Autoimmune Diseases: Symptoms, Diagnosis and Treatment**
*Kyle J. Brenner(Editor)*
2010. ISBN: 978-1-61668-519-5 (E-book)

**Host-Pathogen Interactions: Genetics, Immunology and Physiology**
*Annette W. Barton (Editor)*
2010. ISBN: 978-1-60876-286-6

**Immunotherapy: Activation, Suppression and Treatments**
*Blake C. Facinelli (Editor)*
2010. ISBN: 978-1-61668-585-0

**Immunotherapy: Activation, Suppression and Treatments**
*Blake C. Facinelli (Editor)*
2010. ISBN: 978-1-61668-868-4 (E-book)

**Immunology in Clinic Practice**
*Cagatay Oktenli (Editor)*
2010. ISBN: 978-1-60876-644-4

**Quantitative Immunohistology: Problems and Solutions**
*Anthony S-Y Leong and ,Trishe Y-M Leong*
2010. ISBN: 978-1-61668-261-3

**Lupus Nephritis: Frontiers and Challenges**
*Hussein A. Sheashaa, Tarek M. Abbas, Fatma E. Moustafa, Khaled Mahmoud, Amgad el-Agroudy, Anil Chandraker, Nidyanandh Vadivel, Rashad Hassan, Ashraf M. Bakr, Mohamed Zedan, Noha Tharwat, Wael I. Elkady, Helmut G. Rennke and Mohamed Sobh*
2010. ISBN: 978-1-61668-367-2

**Lupus Nephritis: Frontiers and Challenges**
*Hussein A. Sheashaa, Tarek M. Abbas, Fatma E. Moustafa, Khaled Mahmoud, Amgad el-Agroudy, Anil Chandraker, Nidyanandh Vadivel, Rashad Hassan, Ashraf M. Bakr, Mohamed Zedan, Noha Tharwat, Wael I. Elkady, Helmut G. Rennke and Mohamed Sobh*
2010. ISBN: 378-1-61668-824-0 (E-book)

IMMUNOLOGY AND IMMUNE SYSTEM DISORDERS

# IMMUNOLOGY IN CLINIC PRACTICE

CAGATAY OKTENLI
EDITOR

Nova Science Publishers, Inc.
*New York*

For permission to use material from this book please contact us:
Telephone 631-231-7269; Fax 631-231-8175
Web Site: http://www.novapublishers.com



**LIBRARY OF CONGRESS CATALOGING-IN-PUBLICATION DATA**

Immunology in clinic practice / editor, Cagatay Oktenli.
p. ; cm.
Includes bibliographical references and index.
ISBN 978-1-60876-644-4 (hardcover)
1. Clinical immunology. I. Oktenli, Cagatay.
[DNLM: 1. Allergy and Immunology. 2. Immune System Phenomena. QW 504 I3325 2009]
RC582.I472 2009
616.07'9--dc22

2009044323

*Published by Nova Science Publishers, Inc. † New York*

# DEDICATION

*To Zeki*
*"Truly great friend as you*
*are hard to find,*
*difficult to leave,*
*and impossible to forget"*

*The authors of this book would like to dedicate this work*
*to Dr. Zeki Yeşilova (1968 - 2009),*
*whose unexpected loss is not replaceable.*
*May you rest in peace*
*we miss you lots already*
*August 3, 2009*

# CONTENTS

# PREFACE

*Science is a wonderful thing if one does not have to earn one's living at it.*
*Albert Einstein*

There is a large and rapidly growing body of literature on the immunology in clinic practise. In this book, we have made an effort to brief descriptions of recent immunological developments in clinic practise. This book is not a textbook. All the chapters in the book are independent of each other; each is dedicated to a different clinic. To meet the needs of different readers, all chapters have a similar structure. Though the field of immunology has a wide range of research, we have tried to include the important developments in the book with examples and recent references. References are provided at the end of each chapter. For clinicians, this book provides a broad perspective on immunology, their possible applications and interactions between special clinics, and suggestions about future research topics, which will be helpful to their research. We hope that regardless of your backround whether as an immunologist, internal specialist, surgeon, cardiolog, or a psychiatrist, you will find the book appropriate to your needs.

All the authors are experts in their specific areas. Each chapter reflects their own opinion, comment, experience, and achievements. Also, each author assumes sole responsibility for the general content of their chapters and for all conclusions and citations. They have given much under the tremendous pressures of their many other obligations. As an editor, I greatly appreciate their support, dedication and friendship. Unfortunately, during the submission period of this book, *Dr. Zeki Yeşilova* passed away suddenly due to a massive heart attack on August 3, 2009 at the age of 41. He was a very special man, and he lives on in our hearts and in our memories. We are also most appreciative to the editors of Nova Science Publishers, Inc., for their work in bringing this book to publication. Lastly, most of all my thanks go to my family; my wife, *Gina*, and my son, *Burak*.

Prof. Çağatay Öktenli
Chief, Division of Internal Medicine
GATA Haydarpaşa Training Hospital
İstanbul, Turkey

In: Immunology in Clinic Practice
Editor: Cagatay Oktenli, pp. 3-11

ISBN 978-1-60876-644-4


*Chapter 1*

# CURRENT PERSPECTIVES ON IMMUNOLOGY AND HEPATOLOGY

***Zeki Yeşilova***
Department of Gastroenterology,
Gülhane Military Medical Academy, Ankara, Turkey

## ABSTRACT

Autoimmune hepatitis, primary biliary cirrhosis and primary sclerosing cholangitis are the three major immune-mediated liver diseases. Autoimmune hepatitis is a disease of unknown etiology, entailing progressive destruction of the hepatic parenchyma. The autoimmune aetiology of autoimmune hepatitis is generaly accepted. Primary biliary cirrhosis is a chronic, slowly progressive, autoimmune, cholestatic liver disease that affects predominantly middle-aged women. Primary biliary cirrhosis is characterised histologically by damage to, and eventual loss of, the biliary epithelial cells lining small intrahepatic bile ducts. The exact mechanism underlying the pathogenesis of primary biliary cirrhosis remains uncertain, but both cellular and humoral abnormalities have both been noted. The strong association of primary sclerosing cholangitis with a series of autoimmune diseases underscores the role of immunological alterations in the pathophysiology of the disease.

**Keywords:** autoimmune hepatitis; primary biliary cirrhosis; primary sclerosing cholangitis; antimitochondrial antibodies; anti-liver kidney microsome type 1

## INTRODUCTION

The liver is continuously exposed to large antigenic load that includes pathogens tumur cells, toxins and dietary antigens. A loss of tolerance aganist its own antigens may result autoimmune hepatitis (AIH) [1]. The autoimmune hypothesis of AIH is that individuals with agenetic predisposition may suffer from an autoimmune proces triggered by autoreactive T-cells which leads to chronic hepatitis. The presense of lymphoctes in the liver is considered to be associated with pathogenesis of AIH. Primary biliary cirrhosis (PBC) is a chronic, slowly progressive, autoimmune, cholestatic liver disease that affects predominantly middle-aged women. PBC is characterised histologically by damage to, and eventual loss of, the small intrahepatic bile ducts. The factors that determine individual risk of disease progression remain unclear. Primary sclerosing cholangitis (PSC) is a chronic cholestatic liver disease characterized by fibrosing inflammatory destruction of the intrahepatic and/or extrahepatic bile ducts. PSC is associated with a 10% to 20% lifetime risk for the development of cholangiocarcinoma.

## AUTOIMMUNE HEPATITIS

Autoimmune hepatitis (AIH) is a self-perpetuating inflammation of the liver [2,3]. Diagnostic criteria for AIH, the International Autoimmune Hepatitis Group first formulated in 1993 [4]. Anti-smooth-muscle antibodies are characteristic antibody for type 1 AIH. Anti-nuclear antibodies are also reported in 70% of type 1 AIH patients [4,5]. On the other hand, anti-liver kidney microsome type 1 (LKM1) is specific antibody for Type 2 AIH [5]. It has been suggested that this autoantibody is directed against the cytochrome P450 2D6 (CYP2D6) [6].

Multiple susceptibility alleles can encode the same or similar sequence in AIH [7,8]. The clinical phenotype can be modified by genetic polymorphisms that affect the immune-mediated mechanisms [7]. Cytotoxic lymphocytes can be directed against normal liver tissue. These can perpetuate the immune response and extend the injury. The antigen recognition sites of the autoreactive $CD8^+$ and $CD4^+$ T cells are limited. Thus, these restrictions suggest that the repertoire of driving antigens is small in AIH. It has been also suggested that the apoptotic pathway for immunocyte deletion is defective in AIH [9]. On the other hand, the counter-regulatory cytokine profile is also defective in AIH. This can contribute to the clonal expansion of liver-infiltrating cytotoxic T cells. These defects may reflect the failure of T-regulatory cells to modulate $CD8^+$ T-cell proliferation and production of cytokines [10]. In this way, they suppress IFN-γ production, whereas they increase secretion of IL-4, IL-10, and TGF-β. T-regulatory cells exert a direct suppressive effect on the immune response by modifying the cytokine profile [11]. This may also be modulated by genetic factors [12]. Corticosteroids can reconstitute T-regulatory cell function in AIH.

A characteristic immunogenetic phenotype consisting of HLA A1, B8, DR3 or DR4 is reported in a majority of cases. HLA DRB1*13 has also been associated with autoimmune hepatitis in 54% [13-15].

Finally, although exact pathogenic mechanisms have not yet been delineated, AIH is a manifestation of dysregulated immunoreaction of the suppressor T cells [16]. Auto-antibodies seen in patients with AIH do have an immense diagnostic importance, but their role in the pathogenesis is unclear [17].

## Primary Biliary Cirrhosis

Primary biliary cirrhosis (PBC) is a chronic, slowly progressive, autoimmune, cholestatic liver disease [18-20]. Classical triad for the disease are antimitochondrial antibodies (AMA) in serum, cholestatic indices and liver histology compatible with PBC. AMA is negative in approximately 10% of PBC patients. These patients should be carefully evaluated for the presence of PBC by cholangiography or liver biopsy [18]. PBC have a female predominance [21]. PBC affects individuals of all ethnic origin and accounts for 0.6~2.0% of deaths from cirrhosis worldwide [22]. Its prevalence is estimated to be between 6.7 and 940 cases per million-population [23-25]. PBC is also more frequent in relatives of affected individuals [26-28]. Recent data suggest that X-chromosome monosomy in lymphoid cells is common in women with PBC [29].

PBC is referred to as a "model autoimmune disease" because not only the presence of autoantibodies in the sera was identified but also the antigen specificity of the autoreactive response was characterized for the disease [30]. PBC is regarded as an autoimmune disorder and, in its pathogenesis, immune mediated destruction of epithelial cells of bile duct is proposed [31,32]. The recruited T cells, neutrophils, or monocytes can act as part of a protective response against biliary infections or as participants in the inflammation of the bile ducts [32]. $CD4^+$ and $CD8^+$ T cells are present in portal and periportal areas as well as the peripheral blood in the majority of patients with PBC [33]. Furthermore, abnormal suppressor T-cell activity has been reported in asymptomatic first-degree relatives of people with the disease [34]. On the other hand, PBC exhibit clustering with various autoimmune disorders, both within individuals and family [35]. In this way, regulatory T cells were found to be decreased in PBC [12].

Recently, it has been suggested that a significant rise in the percentage and number in peripheral blood and liver of NK cells in PBC [36]. Innate immunity is also activated in PBC patients [37]. It has been reported that exposure of peripheral blood mononuclear cells of these patients to non-methylated oligonucleotides results in the production of various cytokines such as IL-1β, TNF-α, IL-6 and IL-8 [37]. Moreover, Th1 cytokine predominance plays an important role in recruitment of memory T-cells in PBC and may be responsible for the progressive bile duct damage [38,39]. Indeed, peripheral blood mononuclear cells in PBC patients preferentially synthesize Th1 cytokines [40,41]. Furthermore, biliary epithelial cell stimulation with lipopolysaccharide increases production of TNF-α [42]. In addition to AMA, PBC sera can present other disease-specific autoantibodies such as ANA and anti-centromere antibodies [43].

## Primary Sclerosing Cholangitis

Primary sclerosing cholangitis (PSC) is a chronic cholestatic liver disease characterized by fibrosing inflammatory destruction of the intrahepatic and/or extrahepatic bile ducts [44-51]. The majority of cases (75%) occur in association with inflammatory bowel disease (IBD) such as ulcerative colitis and Crohn's disease [45, 48, 49]. PSC can affect both large and small bile ducts [46]. The mean age at diagnosis is 40 years and men are affected about two times more than women [47].

Accumulating evidence suggest that the immunological alterations may play an important role in the pathophysiology of the disease [51]. It has been suggested that the liver is infiltrated with activated mucosal T cells in PSC [52]. In addition, these T cells are long-lived memory cells capable of being activated to secrete pro-inflammatory cytokines [53].

Specific autoantibodies such as antineutrophil cytoplasmatic antibodies (p-ANCA), anticolon antibodies, antineutrophil nuclear antibodies can be found in patients with PSC with a high frequency but lacking in diagnostic specificity [54-62]. However, anti-mitochondrial auto-antibodies (AMA), anti-nuclear auto-antibodies (ANA), and anti-smooth muscle auto-antibodies (ASMA) were reported a lower frequency [56-62]. Hyper-γ-globulinemia is found in 30% of patients, an increase of IgM in 40-50% [57]. The biliary epithelial cells appear to be the target of immune-mediated injury. Therefore, on bile ducts, dense infiltrations with activated T cells, high local concentrations of pro-inflammatory cytokines and increased HLA expression are common [63].

Although the exact role of immune system alterations in the development, behaviour and progression of the disease is still not clear, many patients of PSC (80%) have circulating immune complexes [64]. Hypergammaglobulinemia, high serum IgM, decreased circulating T cells, increased ratio of CD4:CD8 and decreased $C_3$ are other immunological abnormalities [65,66]. On the other hand, lymphocytic bile duct destruction and an increase of MHC II on biliary epithelial cells were reported at histology, [67,68].

Furthermore, in PSC, a Th1 cytokine predominance has been suggested [69,70]. In this manner, TNF-α and IL-1β levels were found to be high concentrations, whereas IL-2, IL-10 and IFN-γ levels were low in supernatants of liver-infiltrating lymphocytes from PSC patients [71].

## Conclusion

Development of AIH requires a series of events such as viral infection and/or chemical exposure in a suitable environment such as genetic background of susceptibility, female sex and young age [72]. Further clinical and fundamental investigations will be needed before the pathogenesis of AIH is fully understood. There has been a rapid growth in our understanding of the underlying mechanisms of PBC. Using the recombinant cloned antigen as a tool, research has focused on the intrahepatic bile ducts [73]. In this context, future therapeutic efforts in PBC will depend mainly on understanding the nature of these innate immune responses [73]. PSC is a progressive disorder and no curative therapy is available at the current time except liver transplantation [74,75].

## References

[1] Czaja, A.J. (2007) Evolving concepts in the diagnosis, pathogenesis and treatment of autoimmune hepatitis. *Minerva Gastroenterol. Dietol*, 53, 43–78.

[2] Takahashi, H. (2007) Current topics relating to autoimmune hepatitis diagnosis and therapy. *Hepatol. Res*, 37, S510–514.

[3] Czaja, A.J. (2007) Autoimmune hepatitis. Part A: pathogenesis. *Expert Rev Gastroenterol Hepatol*, 1, 113–128.

[4] Johnson, P.J., McFarlane, I.G. (1993) Meeting report: International Autoimmune Hepatitis Group. *Hepatol*, 18, 998–1005.

[5] Krawitt, E.L. (2006) Autoimmune hepatitis. *N. Engl. J. Med*, 354, 54–66.

[6] Manns, M.P., Johnson, E.F., Griffin, K.J., Tan, E.M., Sullivan, K.F. (1989) Major antigen of liver kidney microsomal autoantibodies in idiopathic autoimmune hepatitis is cytochrome P450db1. *J. Clin. Invest*, 83, 1066–1072.

[7] Czaja, AJ. (2005) Diverse manifestations and evolving treatments of autoimmune hepatitis. *Minerva Gastroenterol. Dietol*, 51, 313–333.

[8] Czaja, A.J. (2005) Current concepts in autoimmune hepatitis. *Ann. Hepatol*, 4, 6–24.

[9] Ichiki, Y., Aoki, C.A., Bowlus, C.L., Shimoda, S., Ishibashi, H., Gershwin, M.E. (2005) T cell immunity in autoimmune hepatitis. *Autoimmun. Rev*, 4, 315–321.

[10] Longhi, M.S., Ma, Y., Mitry, R.R., Bogdanos, D.P., Heneghan, M., Cheeseman, P., Mieli-Vergani, G., Vergani, D. (2005) Effect of CD4+ CD25+ regulatory T-cells on CD8 T-cell function in patients with autoimmune hepatitis. *J. Autoimmun*, 25, 63–71.

[11] Longhi, M.S., Mitry, R.R., Samyn, M., Scalori, A., Hussain, M.J., Quaglia, A., Mieli-Vergani, G., Ma, Y., Vergani, D. (2009) Vigorous activation of monocytes in juvenile autoimmune liver disease escapes the control of regulatory T-cells. *Hepatology*, 50, 130-142.

[12] Lan, R.Y., Cheng, C., Lian, Z.X., Tsuneyama, K., Yang, G.X., Moritoki, Y., Chuang, Y.H., Nakamura, T., Saito, S., Shimoda, S., Tanaka, A., Bowlus, C.L., Takano, Y., Ansari, A.A., Coppel, R.L., Gershwin, M.E. (2006) Liver-targeted and peripheral blood alterations of regulatory T cells in primary biliary cirrhosis. *Hepatology*, 43, 729–737.

[13] Czaja, A.J., Carpenter, H.A., Moore, S.B. (2006) Clinical and HLA phenotypes of type 1 autoimmune hepatitis in North American patients outside DR3 and DR4. *Liver Int*, 26, 552–558.

[14] Czaja, A.J., Carpenter, H.A., Moore, S.B. (2008) HLA DRB1*13 as a risk factor for type 1 autoimmune hepatitis in North American patients. *Dig. Dis. Sci*, 53, 522–528.

[15] Lohse, A.W., Hennes, E. (2007) Diagnostic criteria for autoimmune hepatitis. *Hepatol. Res*, 37, S509.

[16] Czaja, A.J. (2001) Understanding the pathogenesis of autoimmune hepatitis. *Am. J. Gastroenterol.*, 96, 1224–1231.

[17] Joshi, M., Khettry, U. (2009) Approach to diagnosis of auto-immune hepatitis. *Indian J. Pathol. Microbiol.*, 52, 297-303.

[18] Kaplan, M.M., Gerschwin, M.E. (2005) Primary biliary cirrhosis. *N Engl. J. Med*, 353, 1261-1273.

[19] Wasilenko, S.T., Mason, G.E., Mason, A.L. (2009) Primary biliary cirrhosis, bacteria and molecular mimicry: what's the molecule and where's the mimic? *Liver Int*, 29, 779-782.

[20] Harada, K., Shimoda, S., Sato, Y., Isse, K., Ikeda, H., Nakanuma, Y. (2009) Periductal interleukin-17 production in association with biliary innate immunity contributes to the pathogenesis of cholangiopathy in primary biliary cirrhosis. *Clin. Exp. Immunol*, 157, 261-270.

[21] Dahlan, Y., Smith, L., Simmons, D., Jewell, L.D., Wanless, I., Heathcote, E.J., Bain, V.G. (2003) Pediatric-onset primary biliary cirrhosis. *Gastroenterology*, 125, 1476–1479.

[22] Kaplan, M.M. (1987) Primary biliary cirrhosis. *N. Engl. J. Med*, 26, 521–528.

[23] James, O.F., Bhopal, R., Howel, D., Gray, J., Burt, A.D., Metcalf, J.V. (1999) Primary biliary cirrhosis once rare, now common in the United Kingdom? *Hepatology*, 30, 390–394.

[24] Kim, W.R., Lindor, K.D., Locke, G.R. 3rd, Therneau, T.M., Homburger, H.A., Batts, K.P., et al. (2000) Epidemiology and natural history of primary biliary cirrhosis in a US community. *Gastroenterology*, 119, 1631–1636.

[25] Selmi, C. (2004) Epidemiology and pathogenesis of primary biliary cirrhosis. *J. Clin. Gastroenterol*, 38, 264–271.

[26] Invernizzi, P. (2005) From bases to basis: linking genetics to causation in primary biliary cirrhosis. *Clin. Gastroenterol. Hepatol*, 3, 401–410.

[27] Jones, D.E., Watt, F.E., Metcalf, J.V., Bassendine, M.F., James, O.F. (1999) Familial primary biliary cirrhosis reassessed: a geographically-based population study. *J. Hepatol*, 30, 402-407.

[28] Semli, C., Mayo, M.J., Bach, N., Ishibashi, H., Invernizzi, P., Gish, R.G. (2004) Primary biliary cirrhosis in monozygotic and dizygotic twins: genetics, epigenetics, and environment. *Gastroenterology*, 127, 485-492.

[29] Invernizzi, P., Miozzo, M., Battezzati, P.M., Bianchi, I., Grati, F.R., Simoni, G. (2004) Frequency of monosomy X in women with primary biliary cirrhosis. *Lancet*, 363, 533-535.

[30] Yeaman, S.J., Kirby, J.A., Jones, D.E. (2000) Autoreactive responses to pyruvate dehydrogenase complex in the pathogenesis of primary biliary cirrhosis. *Immunol. Rev.*, 174, 238-249.

[31] Kumagi, T., Heathcote, E.J. (2008) Primary biliary cirrhosis. *Orphanet J. Rare Dis.*, 3, 1–17.

[32] Wu, C.T., Davis, P.A., Luketic, V.A., Gershwin, M.E. (2004) A review of the physiological and immunological functions of biliary epithelial cells: targets for primary biliary cirrhosis, primary sclerosing cholangitis and drug-induced ductopenias. *Clin. Dev. Immunol.*, 11, 205–213.

[33] Palmer, J.M., Kirby, J.A., Jones, D.E.J. (2002) The immunology of primary biliary cirrhosis: the end of the beginning? *Clin. Exp. Immunol.,* 129, 191-197.

[34] Hashimoto, E., Lindor, K.D., Homburger, H.A., et al. (1993) Immunohistochemical characterization of hepatic lymphocytes in primary biliary cirrhosis in comparison with primary sclerosing cholangitis and autoimmune chronic active hepatitis. *Mayo Clin. Proc*, 68, 1049–1055.

[35] Hohenester, S., Oude-Elferink, R.P., Beuers, U. (2009) Primary biliary cirrhosis. *Semin. Immunopathol.,* 31, 283-307.

[36] Chuang, Y.H., Lian, Z.X., Tsuneyama, K., Chiang, B.L., Ansari, A.A., Coppel, R.L., Eric Gershwin, M. (2006) Increased killing activity and decreased cytokine production in NK cells in patients with primary biliary cirrhosis. *J. Autoimmun.,* 26, 232-240.

[37] Mao, T.K., Lian, Z.X., Selmi, C., Ichiki, Y., Ashwood, P., Ansari, A.A., et al. (2005) Altered monocyte responses to defined TLR ligands in patients with primary biliary cirrhosis. *Hepatology,* 42, 802-808.

[38] Harada, K., Nakanuma, Y. (2006) Molecular mechanisms of cholangiopathy in primary biliary cirrhosis. *Med. Mol. Morphol.,* 39, 55-61.

[39] Harada, K., Isse, K., Kamihira, T., Shimada, S., Nakanuma, Y. (2005) Th1 cytokine-induced downregulation of PPARgamma in human biliary cells relates to cholangitis in primary biliary cirrhosis. *Hepatology,* 41, 1328-1338.

[40] Sekiya, H., Komatsu, T., Isono, E., Furukawa, M., Matsushima, S., Yamaguchi, N. et al. (1999) Decrease in the prevalence of IL-4-producing CD4 T cells in patients with advanced stage of primary biliary cirrhosis. *Am. J. Gastroenterol.*, 94, 3589-3594.

[41] Nagano, T., Yamamoto, K., Matsumoto, S., Okamoto, R., Tagashira, M., Ibuki, N., et al. (1999) Cytokine profile in the liver of primary biliary cirrhosis. *J. Clin. Immunol.*, 19, 422-427.

[42] Harada, K., Ohira, S., Isse, K., Ozaki, S., Zen, Y., Sato, Y. et al. (2003) Lipopolysaccharide activates nuclear factor-kappaB through toll-like receptors and related molecules in cultured biliary epithelial cells. *Lab. Invest.,* 83, 1657-1667.

[43] Lleo, A., Invernizzi, P., Mackay, I.R., Prince, H., Zhong, R.Q., Gershwin, M.E. (2008) Etiopathogenesis of primary biliary cirrhosis. *World J. Gastroenterol.,* 14, 3328-3337.

[44] Mattalia, A., Quaranta, S., Leung, P.S., Bauducci, M., Van de Water, J., Calvo, P.L. (1998) Characterization of antimitochondrial antibodies in health adults. *Hepatology*, 27, 656-661.

[45] Tischendorf, J.J., Hecker, H., Kruger, M., Manns, M.P., Meier, P.N. (2007) Characterization, outcome, and prognosis in 273 patients with primary sclerosing cholangitis: A single center study. *Am. J. Gastroenterol*, 102, 107–114.

[46] Talwalkar, J.A., Lindor, K.D. (2005) Primary sclerosing cholangitis. *Inflamm. Bowel Dis*, 11, 62-72.

[47] LaRusso, N.F., Shneider, B.L., Black, D., Gores, G.J., James, S.P., Doo, E., Hoofnagle, J.H. (2006) Primary sclerosing cholangitis: summary of a workshop. *Hepatology*, 44, 746–764.

[48] Olsson, R., Danielsson, A., Jarnerot, G., Lindstrom, E., Loof, L., Rolny, P., et al. (1991) Prevalence of primary sclerosing cholangitis in patients with ulcerative colitis. *Gastroenterology*, 100, 1319-1323.

[49] Kaplan, M.M. (1997) Toward better treatment of primary sclerosing cholangitis. *N. Engl. J. Med*, 336, 719–721.

[50] Schrumpf, E., Fausa, O., Elgjo, K., Kolmannskog, F. (1988) Hepatobiliary complications of inflammatory bowel disease. *Semin. Liver Dis*, 8, 201-220.

[51] Lee, Y.M., Kaplan, M.M. (1995) Primary sclerosing cholangitis. *N. Engl. J. Med*, 332, 924-933.

[52] Mora, J.R., Bono, M.R., Manjunath, N., Weninger, W., Cavanagh, L.L., Rosemblatt, M., et al. (2000) Selective imprinting of gut-homing T cells by Peyer's patch dendritic cells. *Nature*, 424, 88-93.

[53] Eksteen, B., Grant, A.J., Miles, A., Curbishley, S.M., Lalor, P.F., Hubscher, S.G., et al. (2004) Hepatic endothelial CCL25 mediates the recruitmentof CCR9+ gut-homing lymphocytes to the liver in primary sclerosing cholangitis. *J. Exp. Med.,* 200, 1511-1517.

[54] Steckman, M., Drossman, D.A., Lesesne, H.R. (1984) Hepatobiliary disease that precedes ulcerative colitis. *J. Clin. Gastroenterol*, 6, 425-428.

[55] Lee, Y.M., Kaplan, M.M. (2002) Management of primary sclerosing cholangitis. *Am. J. Gastroenterol*, 97, 528–534.

[56] Mulder, A.H., Horst, G., Haagsma, E.B., Limburg, P.C., Kleibeuker, J.H., Kallenberg, C.G. (1993) Prevalence and characterization of neutrophil cytoplasmic antibodies in autoimmune liver diseases. *Hepatology*, 17, 411-417..

[57] Bansi, D., Chapman, R., Fleming, K. (1996) Antineutrophil cytoplasmic antibodies in chronic liver diseases: prevalence, titre, specificity and IgG subclass. *J. Hepatol*, 24, 581-586.

[58] Mehal, W.Z., Lo, Y.M., Wordsworth, B.P., Neuberger, J.M., Hubscher, S.C., Fleming, K.A. (1994) HLA DR4 is a marker for rapid disease progression in primary sclerosing cholangitis. *Gastroenterology*, 106, 160-167.

[59] Duerr, R.H., Targan, S.R., Landers, C.J., Larusso, N.F., Lindsay, K.L., Wiesner, R.H. (1991) Neutrophil cytoplasmic antibodies: a link between primary sclerosing cholangitis and ulcerative colitis. *Gastroenterology*, 100, 1385-1391.

[60] Zauli, D., Schrumpf, E., Crespi, C., Cassani, F., Fausa, O., Aadland, E. (1987) An autoantibody profile in primary sclerosing cholangitis. *J. Hepatol*, 5, 14-18.

[61] Snook, J.A., Chapman, R.W., Fleming, K., Jewell, D.P. (1989) Anti-neutrophil nuclear antibody in ulcerative colitis, Crohn's disease and primary sclerosing cholangitis. *Clin. Exp. Immunol*, 76, 30-33.

[62] Wiesner, R.H., Larusso, N.F., Ludwig, J., Dickson, E.R. (1985) Comparison of the clinicopathologic features of primary sclerosing cholangitis and primary biliary cirrhosis. *Gastroenterology*, 88, 108-114.

[63] O'Mahony, C.A., Vierling, J.M. (2006) Etiopathogenesis of primary sclerosing cholangitis. *Semin. Liver Dis*, 26, 3–21.

[64] Grant, A.J., Lalor, P.F., Hubscher, S.G., Briksin, M., Adams, D.H. (2001) MAdCAM-1 expressed in chronic inflammatory liver disease supports mucosal lymphocyte adhesion to hepatic endothelium (MAdCAM-1 in chronic inflammatory liver disease). *Hepatology*, 33, 1065-1072.

[65] Bodenheimer, H.C. Jr, Larusso, N.F., Thayer, W.R. Jr, Charland, C., Staples, P.J., Ludwig, J. (1983) Elevated circulating immune complexes in primary sclerosing cholangitis. *Hepatology*, 3, 150-154.

[66] Lindor, K.D., Wiesner, R.H., Katzmann, J.A., Larusso, N.F., Beaver, S.J. (1987) Lymphocyte subsets in primary sclerosing cholangitis. *Dig. Dis. Sci*, 32, 720-725.

[67] Brinch, L., Teisberg, P., Schrumpf, E., Akesson, I. (1982) The in vivo metabolism of C3 in hepatobiliary disease associated with ulcerative colitis. *Scand. J. Gastroenterol*, 17, 523-527.

[68] Ludwig, J., Barham S.S., Larusso, N.F., Elveback, L.R., Wiesner, R.H., McCall, J.T. (1981) Morphologic features of chronic hepatitis associated with primary sclerosing cholangitis and chronic ulcerative colitis. *Hepatology*, 1, 632-640.

[69] Aron, J.H., Bowlus, C.L. (2009) The immunobiology of primary sclerosing cholangitis. *Semin. Immunopathol.*, 31, 383-397.

[70] Aoki, C.A., Dawson, K., Kenny, T.P., Gershwin, M.E., Bowlus, C.L. (2006) Gene expression by PBMC in primary sclerosing cholangitis: evidence for dysregulation of immune mediated genes. *Clin. Dev. Immunol.*, 13, 265-271.

[71] Bo, X., Broome, U., Remberger, M., Sumitran-Holgersson, S. (2001) Tumour necrosis factor alpha impairs function of liver derived T lymphocytes and natural killer cells in patients with primary sclerosing cholangitis. *Gut*, 49, 131-141.

[72] Béland, K., Lapierre, P., Alvarez, F. (2009) Influence of genes, sex, age and environment on the onset of autoimmune hepatitis. *World J. Gastroenterol*, 15, 1025-1034.

[73] Semli, C., Lleo, A., Pasini, S., Zuin, M., Gershwin, M.E. (2009) Innate immunity and primary biliary cirrhosis. *Curr. Mol. Med*, 9, 45-51.

[74] Björnsson, E. (2009) Management of primary sclerosing cholangitis. *Minerva Gastroenterol. Dietol*, 55, 163-172.

[75] LaRusso, N.F., Shneider, B.L., Black, D., Gores, C.J., James, S.P., Doo, E., Hoofnagle, J.H. (2006) Primary sclerosing cholangitis: Summary of a workshop. *Hepatology,* 44, 746-764.

In: Immunology in Clinic Practice
Editor: Cagatay Oktenli, pp. 13-24

ISBN 978-1-60876-644-4


*Chapter 2*

# Overview of Recent Immunological Studies in Obstetrics and Gynecology Clinics

***Murat Dede and Müfit Cemal Yenen***
Department of Obstetric and Gynecology;
Gülhane Military Medical Academy, Ankara, Turkey

## Abstract

Maternal and fetal tissues protect fetus in many ways in utero. Especially, it is well known that amniotic fluid has bacteriostatic properties and amnion cells produce b-defensins. Babies have a high level of maternal IgG at birth because maternal IgG can cross the placenta. They also acquire IgA (and some IgG) postnatally from breast milk; however these remain in the gut lumen. In all species maternal IgG, IgA are important both locally and systemically in protecting the neonate during the development of its own immune system. Furthermore, humoral immune system and T helper (Th) 2 cytokine production are enhanced, whereas cell-mediated immune functions and Th1 cytokine profile are suppressed during pregnancy. In postpartum period, Th1/Th2 cytokine profiles reverse.

**Keywords:** reproduction; pregnancy; maternal fetal immunology; immunologically mediated abortion; preeclampsia; endometriosis

## Introduction

The immune system depends on white blood cells, which play a key role in protecting the body from invasion by pathogenic microorganisms, and disease, particularly cancers. There are two main brances (adaptive and innate) immunity [1, 2]. Innate immunity recognizes the molecular patterns of pathogens by using the genetic memory, while adaptive immunity builds an antigen specific response [1]. Consequently, effective immune response depends on interplay and regulation between adaptive and innate immunity [1]. Polymorphonuclear leukocytes (PMNL), monocytes, macrophages and natural killer (NK) cells are primary effector cells in innate immunity [3,4]. It is very important to understand the underlying mechanisms of fetal, maternal and fetomaternal immunological changes in pregnancy. Moreover, recurrent miscarriages and preterm labors are in the immunological field.

# 1. Normal Pregnancy

Classically, the neonatal elements such as skin, epithelial cells, mucous membranes, endothelial cells and secretions of the innate immune response include non-specific physical immunological barriers to entry of pathogens [1, 5-9]. Thus, in utero, the fetus is protected by these maternal and fetal layers [10-12]. In addition, amnion cells produce antimicrobial b-defensins and amniotic fluid has additional bacteriostatic properties [1].

The number of natural killer cells in the uterus increase in early pregnancy [4]. The origin of uterine NK cells are not known yet. It is possible that they may arise by proliferation and differentiation of NK cell progenitors in utero. In this way, proliferation of this kind of NK cells in late-secretory endometrium and decidua has been shown [13,14]. This is under the control of the sex steroids such as estrogen and progesterone. Moreover, proliferation and differentiation of uterine NK cells can also be induced by IL-15 [13].

Human leukocyte antigen (HLA)-G is a member of the family of nonclassical HLA class I molecules [2] and fetal tissues expresses HLA-G specifically [14,15,18]. It has been demonstrated that *in vitro*-fertilized pre-implantation embryos released soluble HLA-G1 and/or HLAG5, whereas clinical pregnancy was obtained only if soluble HLA-G molecules were present in *in vitro*-growing embryos [3]. Moreover, peripheral blood soluble HLA-G levels were reported to be significantly higher in pregnant women than non-pregnants [3]. Moreover, extravillous cytotrophoblast in first-trimester period expresses both HLA-G protein and messenger ribonucleic acid (mRNA), while villous cytotrophoblast and syncytiotrophoblast in first-trimester are positive for HLA-G mRNA but negative for HLA-G protein [3]. On the other hand, the extravillous cytotrophoblast HLA-G expression increases, whereas the presence of syncytiotrophoblast HLA-G mRNA decreases in the term placenta [3]. Furthermore, a polymorphism in the 3' untranslated region of HLA-G exon 8 is related with the success of in vitro fertilisation [17].

Adaptive/acquired immune system exhibits two main characteristics [19-31]:

1. Memory: The acquired/adaptive immune system will respond more effectively to a secondary exposure of any given antigen. This results in a protective response.
2. Specificity: The specificity of the immune system allows it to selectively recognize different foreign antigens, while maintaining tolerance to an equally diverse panel of self antigens. Failure of this system results in increased susceptibility to autoimmune disorders.

Babies have a high level of maternal IgG at birth because, in humans, maternal IgG can cross the placenta . They also acquire IgA (and some IgG) postnatally from breast milk; however these remain in the gut lumen [28]. In all species maternal IgG, IgA are important both locally and systemically in protecting the neonate during the development of its own immune system.

## 2. MATERNAL FETAL IMMUNOLOGY

Normally, hematopoiesis takes place in the bone marrow in adults, but no bone exists in the embryo and until 12 weeks' gestation. The long bones are not of sufficient size to develop a marrow cavity that can support hematopoiesis in this period. Prior to this time, the first hematopoietic cells are developed extra-embryonically in the yolk sac as early as day 16 of development. Hematopoiesis in the yolk sac is primitive and restricted to erytropoiesis [32]. Cells with a characteristic primitive hematopoietic behaviour are found in the ventral endotelium of the dorsal aorta late in the 4$^{th}$ week of gestation and disappear in the 6$^{th}$ week of gestation. Besides the major cell lineage erythrocytes, cells from the granulocytic and megakaryocytic lineages are found in the fetal liver. The final site for hematopoiesis during fetal development is the bone marrow. Bone marrow stroma appears in week 9-10 of gestation and about three weeks later, active hematopoiesis in the bone marrow begins. At week 22 of gestation all cell lines are represented in the bone marrow, indicating that the fetal bone marrow does not become the major hematopoietic organ until late in the 2$^{nd}$ or early in the 3$^{rd}$ trimester [33].

The womb provides a physical barrier between the fetus and the outside world so The human fetus is protected from most pathogens and the maternal immunity guards against infections of the mother and fetus. If this arrangement would be sufficient, it is possible that maturation of the fetal immune system could be delayed until the 3$^{rd}$ trimester of pregnancy. However, the fetus could need a functioning immune system earlier than that e.g. when the mother's immune system has failed to clear an infection and when the physical barrier to the outer world is disrupted. Previously, the early 2$^{nd}$ trimester fetus has been described as pre-immune, i.e. unable to mount an immunological response against donor cells. Recently, in the fetus, it is well known that lymphocytes are found at the end of the 1$^{st}$ trimester. Furthermore, half of the cells in the fetal thymus express common T-cell surface phenotypes in the three months of pregnancy [33]. Moreover, T-cell can respond to allogeneic cells in *in vitro* from the 2$^{nd}$ to 3$^{rd}$ gestational months [33]. Clinically successful outcomes after in-utero transplantations have only until recently been achieved in cases of immunodeficiency such as bare lymphocyte syndrome and severe combined immune deficiency cases. In fetuses with hemoglobinopathies (sickle cell disease and thalassemia major), fetal liver cells are rejected. Thus, the fetal immunity plays a crucial role in the success or failure of in-utero transplantations.

Human mesenchymal stem cells (MSCs) were first identified in postnatal bone marrow and later in other human adult tissues, including skin, muscle, connective tissue, adipose tissue, perichondrium and trabecular bone [34-36]. But there is a discussion subject that the quantity of MSCs in term cord blood and peripheral blood. Some groups have identified them in term cord blood; peripheral blood and growth factor-mobilised peripheral blood stem cells (PBSCs), whereas other has not. MSCs can also be isolated from several fetal tissues, such as human 1$^{st}$ trimester blood, bone marrow and liver and from human 2$^{nd}$ trimester kidney, bone marrow, liver, lung, spleen, pancreas, blood, brain and amniotic fluid. MSCs is found among 3000 nucleated cells and frequency declined with advancing gestation in 1$^{st}$ trimester fetal blood [35]. The decrease of circulating MSCs in fetal blood during gestation and the higher frequency of MSCs in the 2$^{nd}$ trimester bone marrow might be related to their migration from one hematopoietic site to another in the developing fetus. This is supported by the detection of maximal numbers of fibroblast colony-forming units in murine fetal liver, spleen and bone marrow at the time hematopoietic begins at each site, suggesting the existence of a stromal stem cell migration.

## 3. Pregnancy and Autoimmunity

Hormonal factors linked to gender and reproductive status is involved in regulating the onset of many autoimmune disorders [37-41]. Systemic lupus erythematosus (SLE) primarily affects women in the reproductive years [42]. Rheumatoid arthritis is also more common in women, but, in contrast to SLE, the highest incidence is at menopause. Interestingly, in women who have any rheumatic diseases, the risk of repeated fetal loss, intrauterine growth restriction, and preterm birth remains higher than in the general population [37-41]. On the other hand, pregnancy-related changes in autoimmune disorders reveal the most compelling evidence that hormonal factors play a crucial role in regulating the expression of these disorders [38]. RA, in contrast to SLE, commonly flares in the postpartum period and remits during pregnancy. It is well known that humoral immunity and Th2 cytokine production are enhanced, whereas cell-mediated immune functions and Th1 cytokine profile are suppressed during pregnancy [43]. However, these profiles reverse in the postpartum period.

## 4. Immunologically Mediated Abortion

Since the fetus and placenta are immunologically different from the mother, immunological factors may play a role in the etiology of recurrent miscarriage [44-46]. In this way, as the fetus and placenta are semi-allogenic to the mother, altered expression of the class I HLA molecules has been postulated to play a role in the etiology of recurrent miscarriage [47,48]. It seems likely that this adaptation system depends on spesific interructions between major histocompability complex (MHC) antigen expression target cells and T–cell receptor expressing lymphocytes [47,48].

Classically, three or more consecutive pregnancy losses is called recurrent miscarriage (RM) [49-52]. RM is multifactorial and in at least 50% of causes, cause is unknown most important cause of RM is cytogenetic abnormalities reported between 35 % - 55% of causes. The antiphospholipid syndrome is the most common of immunologic causes of RM. Moreover, increased frequencies of protrombin G20210A mutations and factor ulerden have been reported in RM [50]. On the other hand, decreased Th2 pattern to trophoblastic and placental antigens was also reported in RM.

Normally, IL-10, an important anti-inflammatory cytokine, is considered crucial in normal pregnancy [53,54]. IL-10 upregulates the HLA-G expression of cytotrophoblasts during pregnancy [51] and it protects the fetus from rejection. IL-10 has considerable regulatory effects against pro-inflammatory cytokines (TNF-α and IFN-γ). In RM, mitogen activated mononuclear cells and maternal decidual T cells show reduced IL-10 expression [53]. Genetic polymorphism related with production of IL-10 may also play a role in RM [50].

In RM, there might be a role of normal intramural flora or endotoxin derived from bacteria. In this way, the activated immunity during pregnancy also modulates the immune response against endotoxins [55]. In experimental studies, it has been also demonstrated that human placental lactogen increases significantly CD14 expression on monocytes [56,57]. On the other hand, bacterial products, proinflammatory cytokines (IL-1β, TNF-α) and other inflammatory mediators (PGE2) originating from periodontal tissues, may affect tissues distant from oral cavity. In this manner, periodontal disease of the mother is associated with low birth weight in newborns [58].

## 5. Preeclampsia and Immunology

Preeclampsia (PE) is a disorder of gestation characterized by proteinuria and hypertension. PE is an important cause of both maternal and perinatal morbidity and mortality. The symptoms normally develop after $5^{th}$ month of gestation and disappear within 7-10 days after delivery. Cases of PE still puzzle us with it's complexity of pathophysiology. Some etiological factors such as poor placentation, endothelial dysfunction, oxidative stress, placental hypoxia, excessive maternal inflammation, poor angiogenesis and renin-angiotensin system dysfunction, immunologic, genetic, and/or environmental factors etc. have been proposed [59-75]. Colbern and Main in 1991 redefined the conceptual framework of reproductive immunology as maternal-placental tolerance instead of maternal-fetal tolerance [62]. Recently, pathophysiology of PE is focused on defective trophoblast invasion and maladaptation of immune responses [60]. In this manner, the embryo in early development divides into two groups of cells, an internal, the inner cell mass and external layer, the embryonic trophoblast that becomes trophoblast cells and later the placenta. The cells from the placenta are the only part of the fetus to interact directly with the mother's cells. Thus, the fetus itself has no direct contact with maternal cells. Normally, implantation is the process by which blastocyts becomes intimately connected with the maternal endometrium/decidua.

There are some immunological mechanisms which prevent the fetal rejection by the maternal immunity, although these are not well established yet [59-75]. The proposed theories can be classified in five ideas: (i) suppression of the maternal immune system during gestation, (ii) a mechanical barier affect of trophoblast, (iii) the lack of trophoblast MHC class I molecules, (iv) local immune supression, and (v) cytokine shift. Varied degrees of deviation from the normal regulated immune system may lead to complications of pregnancy.

Epidemiological evidence seems to indicate that PE appears more commonly in the first conception. Therefore, multiparity is a protective effect for the development of PE. These findings demonstrate that paternal antigen-spesific tolerance is induced by memory T cells during the first gestation and these memory T cells quickly expand the tolerance in the next pregnancies. Expanded paternal-spesific tolerance decrease the risk of PE. During normal pregnancy, immune cells express these activating markers suggesting that the innate immune system is already activated. However, the adaptive immune system, including T cells and B cells does not express activation markers. The immune response dramatically changes in PE. Neutrophils, monocytes and lymphocytes are excessively activated [66].

It is well known that the immune response is controlled via the HLA area on choromosome 6. Placental trophoblasts express primarily the non-classical Class I B antigens.

This trophoblastic expression is likely to protect the fetus from rejection. In this way, several HLA alleles are involved in the pathogenesis of PE and other pregnancy complications. The most prominent one is HLA-G. HLA-G expression is very low or defective in PE [64].

In normal pregnancy, the Th1/Th2 ratio is shifted toward Th2 type reactions and this is thought to facilitate maternal immune tolerance to the fetus [63]. In PE, the balance of Th1 type cytokines to Th2 tye cytokines shifts to Th1 type immunity. Therefore, in circulation, Th1 type cells and cytokines increase, and Th2 type cells and cytokines reduce in PE [25]. Th1 cells and cytokines play major role in induction of inflammation [65].

Trophoblastic apoptotic cells cause massive amount of trophoblastic debris [11]. This debris is released into maternal circulation and activates the macrophages. These macrophages produce immunosuppressive cytokines (IL-10 and TGF-β), and regulate inflammation and Th1 type immunity. In PE, this regulatory process does not work because antigen presenting cells such as macrophages and dentritic cells, phagocyte necrotic trophoblast and produce type 1 cytokines. Increase of TNF-α, IL-12 and IFN-γ augment inflammation. These changes in the immune environment induce apoptosis of extravillous cells resulting in poor placentation in PE.

Many studies have been conducted to reveal that cytokines are involved in pathogenesis of PE. However, the source of these cytokines in circulation of preeclamptic women has not been identified completely yet. Particularly, maternal circulating monocytes, activated immune cells represent a source of cytokines during PE. Some studies showed that plasma levels of TNF-α and IL-1β are increased in PE. On the other hand, conflicting reports on IL-6 and IL-8 show either no difference or increased concentrations. TNF-α may play an important role in the pathogenesis of PE [63]. In pregnancies complicated by PE, IL-12 production may be regulated by elevated IFN-γ and granulocyte-macrophage-colony stimulating factor (GM-CSF). IFN-γ and GM-CSF are produced by hyprstimulated T cells, NK cells or monocytes, which phagocytose aponecrotic trophoblast cell debris. IL-12 production may be regulated by IL-10, TGF-β and $PGE_2$ which are produced by trophoblast, amniotic cells and decidual cells during normal gestation. Immunoregulatory cytokines (TGF-β and IL-10) regulate immunostimulation and inflammation. IL-10 production by peripheral $CD56^+$ NK cells and $CD56^+$ T lymphocytes are anhanced during normal pregnacy. Several studies also demonstrate that IL-10 expression may regulate the process of placentation [67].

## 6. Endometriosis and Immunology

There is evidence for altered cell-mediated and humoral immunity in the pathogenesis of endometriosis [76-78]. Deficient cellular immunity may cause in an inability to recognize the existence of endometrial tissue in abnormal locations. The decreased cytotoxicity to endometrial cells in women with endometriosis is mainly because of a defect in NK activity but is also partially because of a resistance of the endometrium to NK cytotoxicity. It is also likely that the immune system can recognize and eliminate altered or misplaced autologous cells such as ectopic endometrial cells. This mechanism may be operative in most women, preventing the development of endometriosis. In women with endometriosis, it has been demonstrated that functional changes in cells of the immune system [79]. These changes may cause decreased recognition, surveillance and destruction of the misplaced endometrial cells and may facilitate of their implantation and development of endometriosis. On the other hand, secretion of various cytokines by endometrial cells and inflammatory cells into the peritoneal cavity may also lead to recruitment of capillaries, chemoattraction of leukocytes and proliferation of implants. In endometriosis, defective immunosurveillance may cause for the survival of endometrial tissue [80].

## Conclusion

It is well known that reproductive events such as implantation, trofoblast invasion, plasental development and immune protection are all modulated by immune system cells. The immune interaction between fetus and mother is very complex. There are several mechanisms of local and peripheral tolerance induction during gestation. These mechanisms prevent fetal rejection while maintaining strong and active immune surveillance against the pathogens.

## References


[1] Aagaard-Tillery, K.M., Silver, R., Dalton, J. (2006) Immunology of normal pregnancy. *Semin. Fetal.Neonatal. Med*, 11(5):279-95.

[2] Dempsey, P.W., Vaidya, S.A., Cheng, G. (2003) The Art of War: Innate and adaptive immune responses. *Cell Mol. Life Sci*, 60:2604-21.

[3] Karhukorpi, J. (2005) The search for links between immunogenetic factors and recurrent miscarriage. ISBN 951-42-7744-9 http://herkules.oulu.fi/isbn 9514277449.

[4] Moretta, A. (2002) Natural killer cells and pregnancy. *Nat. Rev. Immunol*, 2, 656-663.

[5] Mor, G. (2006) Immunology of pregnancy. Springer, New York ISBN 978-0-387-34944-2

[6] Robertson, S.A. (2007) GM-CSF regulation of embryo development and pregnancy. *Cytokine Growth Fact.Rev*, 18(3-4):287-98.

[7] Reinhard, G., Noll, A., Schlebusch, H., Mallmann, P., Ruecker, A.V. (1998) Shifts in the TH1/TH2 balance during human pregnancy correlate with apoptotic changes. *Biochem. Biophysic Res. Commun*, 245(3):933-8.

[8] Guerin, L.R., Prins, J.R., Robertson, S.A. (2009) Regulatory T-cells and immune tolerance in pregnancy: a new target for infertility treatment? *Hum. Reprod. Update*, 1(1):1-19.

[9] Vigano, P., Cintorino, M., Schatz, F., Lockwood, C.J., Arcuri, F. (2007) The role of macrophage migration inhibitory factor in maintaining the immune privilege at the fetal-maternal interface. *Semin. Immunopathol.*, 29(2):135-50.

[10] Zenclussen, A.C., Schumacher, A., Zenclussen, M.L., Wafula, P., Volk, H.D. (2007) Immunology of pregnancy: cellular mechanisms allowing fetal survival within the maternal uterus. *Expert Rev. Mol. Med.*, 9:1-14.

[11] Riley, J.K. (2008) Trophoblast immune receptors in maternal-fetal tolerance. *Immunol. Invest.*, 37(5-6):395-426.

[12] Trowsdale, J., Betz, A. (2006) Mother's little helpers: mechanisms of maternal-fetal tolerance. *Nat. Immunol.,* 7:241-246.

[13] Santoni, A., Zingoni, A., Cerboni, C., Gismondi, A. (2007) Natural killer (NK) cells from killers to regulators: Distinc features between peripheral blood and decidual NK cells. *Am. J. Reprod. Immunol.,* 58(3):280-8.

[14] Dosiou, C., Giudice, L. (2005) Natural killer cells in pregnancy and recurrent pregnancy loss: endocrine and immunologic perspectives. *Endocrine Rev.,* 26(1):44-62.

[15] Trundley, A., Moffett, A. (2004) Human uterine leukocytes and pregnancy. *Tissue Antigens*, 63, 1-12.

[16] Ferlazzo, G., Pack, M., Thomas, D., Paludan, C., Schmid, D., Strowig, T., et al., (2004) Distinct roles of IL-12 and IL-15 in human natural killer cell activation by dendritic cells from secondary lymphoid organs. *Proc. Natl. Acad*, 101, 16606-11.

[17] Suryanarayana, V., Rao, L., Kanakavalli, M., Padmalatha, V., Deenadayal, M., Singh, L. (2008) Association between novel HLA-G genotypes and risk of recurrent miscarriages: a case-control study in a South Indian population. *Reprod. Sci*, 15, 817-824.

[18] Favier, B., LeMaoult, J., Rouas-Freiss, N., Moreau, P., Menier, C., Carosella, E.D. (2007) Research on HLA-G: an update. *Tissue Antigens,* 69(3):207-11.

[19] Jenkins, S.J., Perona-Wright, G., Macdonald, A.S. (2008) Full development of Th2 immunity requires both innate and adaptive sources of CD154. *J. Immunol*, 180, 8083-8092.

[20] Holt, P.G., Jones, C.A. (2001) The development of the immune system during pregnancy and early life. *Allergy*, 55(8), 688-697.

[21] Garrote, J.A., Arranz, E., Gómez-González, E., León, A.J., Farré, C., Calvo, C., Bernardo, D., et al. (2005) IL6, IL10 and TGFB1 gene polymorphisms in coeliac disease: differences between DQ2 positive and negative patients. *Allergol. Immunopathol*, 33, 245-249.

[22] Fecteau, J.F., Néron, S. (2003) CD40 stimulation of human peripheral B lymphocytes: distinct response from naive and memory cells. *J. Immunol*, 171, 4621-4629.

[23] Cunningham, S.A., Arrate, M.P., Rodriguez, J.M., Bjercke, R.J., Vanderslice, P., Morris, A.P., Brock, T.A. (2000) A novel protein with homology to the junctional adhesion molecule. Characterization of leukocyte interactions. *J. Biol. Chem*, 275, 34750-6.

[24] Aderem, A., Underhill, D.M. (1999) Mechanisms of phagocytosis in macrophages. *Annu. Rev. Immunol*, 17, 593-623.

[25] Beaty, S.R., Rose, C.E. Jr., Sung, S.S. (2007) Diverse and potent chemokine production by lung CD11bhigh dendritic cells in homeostasis and in allergic lung inflammation. *J. Immunol*, 178, 1882.

[26] Meth, M.J., Maibach, H.I. (2006) Current understanding of contrast media reactions and implications for clinical management. *Drug Safety*, 29, 133-141.

[27] Boulanger, E., Fuentes, V., Meignin, V., Mougenot, B., Labaume, S., Gouilleux-Gruart, V., et al. (2006) Polyclonal IgG4 hypergammaglobulinemia associated with plasmacytic lymphadenopathy, anemia and nephropathy. *Ann. Hematol*, 85, 833-840.

[28] Naranatt, P.P., Krishnan, H.H., Svojanovsky, S.R., Bloomer, C., Mathur, S., Chandran, B. (2004) Host gene induction and transcriptional reprogramming in Kaposi's sarcoma-

associated herpesvirus (KSHV/HHV-8)-infected endothelial, fibroblast, and B cells: insights into modulation events early during infection. *Cancer Res*, 64, 72-84.

[29] Marée, A.F., Santamaria, P., Edelstein-Keshet, L. (2006) Modeling competition among autoreactive CD8+ T cells in autoimmune diabetes: implications for antigen-specific therapy. *Int. Immunol*, 2006, 18, 1067-1077.

[30] Bugatti, S., Codullo, V., Caporali, R., Montecucco, C. (2007) B cells in rheumatoid arthritis. *Autoimmun. Rev*, 6, 482-487.

[31] Duhant, X., Suarez, Gonzalez, N., Schandené, L., Goldman, M., Communi, D., Boeynaems, J.M. (2005) Molecular mechanisms of extracellular adenine nucleotides-mediated inhibition of human Cd4(+) T lymphocytes activation. *Purinergic Signal*, 1, 377-381.

[32] Omwandho, C.A., Falconer, J., Gruessner, S.E., Mecha, E., Tumbo-Oeri, A.G., Roberts, T.K., Tinneberg, H.R. (2005) Human placental immunoglobulins show unique re-association patterns with isologous and third party acid treated trophoblast microvesicles in vitro. *East Afr. Med. J*, 82, 290-293.

[33] Padilla-Nash, H.M., Barenboim-Stapleton, L., Difilippantonio, M.J., Ried, T. (2006) Spectral karyotyping analysis of human and mouse chromosomes. *Nat. Protoc*, 1, 3129-3142.

[34] Dezawa, M., Ishikawa, H., Hoshino, M., Itokazu, Y., Nabeshima, Y. (2005) Potential of bone marrow stromal cells in applications for neuro-degenerative, neuro-traumatic and muscle degenerative diseases. *Curr. Neuropharmacol*, 3, 257-266.

[35] Inoue, S., Popp, F.C., Koehl, G.E., Piso, P., Schlitt, H.J., Geissler, E.K., Dahlke, M.H. (2006) Immunomodulatory effects of mesenchymal stem cells in a rat organ transplant model. *Transplantation*, 81, 1589-1595.

[36] Götherstrom, C., Ringden, O., Tammik, C., Zetterberg, E., Westergren, M., Le Blanc, K. (2004) Immunologic properties of human fetal mesenchymal stem cells. *Am. J. Obstet. Gynecol.*, 190(1):239-45.

[37] Yip L, McCluskey J, Sinclair R. (2006) Immunological aspects of pregnancy. *Clin Dermatol.* 24(2):84-7.

[38] Tincani, A., Nuzzo, M., Motta, M., Zati, S., Lojacono, A., Faden, D. (2006) Autoimmunity and pregnancy: autoantibodies and pregnancy in rheumatic diseases. *Ann. N.Y. Acad. Sci*, 1069, 346-352.

[39] Faussett, M.B., Branch, D.W. 2000, Autoimmunity and pregnancy loss. *Semin. Reprod. Med*, 18, 379-392.

[40] Wilder, R.L. (1998) Hormones, pregnancy, and autoimmune diseases. *Ann. N.Y. Acad. Sci.,* 840:45-50.

[41] Ambrosio, P., Lermann, R., Cordeiro, A., Borges, A., Nogueira, I., Serrano, F. (2009) Lupus and pregnancy – 15 Years of experience in a tertiary center. *Clin. Rev. Allergy Immunol.,* Jun 27

[42] Yunis, E.J., Zuniga, J., Romero, V., Yunis, E.J. (2007) Chimerism and tetragametic chimerism in humans: implications in autoimmunity, allorecognition and tolerance. *Immunol. Res*, 38, 213-236.

[43] Karhukorpi, J., Laitinen, T., Karttunen, R., Tiilikainen, A.S. (2001) The functionally important IL-10 promoter polymorphism (-10826 – A) is not a major genetic regulator in recurrent spontaneous abortions. *Mol. Hum. Reprod.*, 7(2):201-3.

[44] Bulletti, C., Flamigni, C., Giacomucci, E. (1996) Reproductive failure due to spontaneous abortion and recurrent miscarriage. *Hum. Reprod. Update,* 2(2):118-36.

[45] Szekeres-Bartho, J., Balasch, J. (2007) Progestagen therapy for recurrent miscarriage. *Hum. Reprod. Update,* 8:1-9.

[46] Bhalla A, Stone PR, Liddell HS, Zanderigo A, Chamley LW. (2006) Comparison of the expression of human leukocyte antigen (HLA)-G and HLA-E in women with normal pregnancy and those with recurrent miscarriage. *Reproduction.* 131(3):583-9

[47] Hanzlikova J, Ulcova-Gallova Z, Malkusova I, Sefrna F, Panzner P. (2009) TH1-TH2 response and the atopy risk in patients with reproduction failure. *Am. J. Reprod. Immunol,* 61, 213-220.

[48] Rubio C, Buendía P, Rodrigo L, Mercader A, Mateu E, Peinado V, Delgado A, Milán M, Mir P, Simón C, Remohí J, Pellicer A. (2009) Prognostic factors for preimplantation genetic screening in repeated pregnancy loss. *Reprod. Biomed. Online,* 18, 687-693.

[49] Giacomucci, E., Bulletti, C., Polli, V., Prefetto, R.A., Flamigni, C. (1994) Immunologically mediated abortion (IMA). *J. Steroid. Biochem. Mol. Biol,* 49, 107-121.

[50] Carp, H.J. (2007) Intravenous immunoglobulin: effect on infertility and recurrent pregnancy loss. *Isr. Med. Assoc. J,* 9, 877-880.

[51] Tien, J.C., Tan, T.Y. (2007) Non-surgical interventions for threatened and recurrent miscarriages. *Singapore Med.. J,* 48, 1074-1090.

[52] Itsekson, A.M., Seidman, D.S., Zolti, M., Lazarov, A., Carp, H.J. (2007) Recurrent pregnancy loss and inappropriate local immune response to sex hormones. *Am. J. Reprod. Immunol,* 57, 160-165.

[53] Stonek, F., Metzenbauer, M., Hafner, E., Philipp, K., Tempfer, C. (2008) Interleukin-10 -1082 G/A promoter polymorphism and pregnancy complications: results of a prospective cohort study in 1,616 pregnant women. *Acta Obstet Gynecol. Scand,* 87, 430-433.

[54] Tayade, C., Black, G.P., Fang, Y., Croy, B.A. (2006) Differential gene expression in endometrium, endometrial lymphocytes, and trophoblasts during successful and abortive embryo implantation. *J. Immunol,* 176, 148-156.

[55] Nagorsen, D., Fetsch, P.A., Abati, A., Marincola, F.M., Panelli, M.C. (2005) Degree of CD14 expression in melanoma infiltrating mononuclear phagocytes. *J. Dermatol. Sci,* 37, 52-54.

[56] Sadauskas, E., Wallin, H., Stoltenberg, M., Vogel, U., Doering, P., Larsen, A., Danscher, G. (2007) Kupffer cells are central in the removal of nanoparticles from the organism. *Part Fibre Toxicol,* 4, 10.

[57] Liu, G., Tsuruta, Y., Gao, Z., Park, Y.J., Abraham, E. (2007) Variant IL-1 receptor-associated kinase-1 mediates increased NF-kappa B activity. *J. Immunol,* 179, 4125-4134.

[58] Gharesi-Fard, B., Zolghadri, J., Foroughinia, L., Tavazoo, F., Samsami, Dehaghani, A. (2007) Effectiveness of leukocyte immunotherapy in primary recurrent spontaneous abortion (RSA). *Iran J. Immunol,* 4, 173-178.

[59] Xia, Y., Zhou, C.C., Ramin, S.M., Kellems, RE. (2007) Angiotensin receptors, autoimmunity, and preeclampsia. *J. Immunol,* 179, 3391-3395.

[60] Clowse, M.E. (2007) Lupus activity in pregnancy. *Rheum. Dis. Clin. North Am,* 33, 237-252.

[61] Kopcow HD, Karumanchi SA. (2007) Angiogenic factors and natural killer (NK) cells in the pathogenesis of preeclampsia. *J Reprod Immunol.* 76(1-2):23-9.

[62] Colbern, G.T., and Main, E.K. (1991) Immunology of the maternal-placental interface in normal pregnancy. *Semin. Perinatol*, 15, 196-205.

[63] Saftlas, A.F., Beydoun, H., Triche, E. (2005) Immunogenetic determinants of preeclampsia and related pregnancy disorders: a systematic review. *Obstet Gynecol*, 106, 162-172.

[64] Redman, C.W., Sargent, I.L. (2005) Latest advances in understanding preeclampsia. *Science*, 308, 1592-1594.

[65] Darmochwal-Kolarz, D., Saito, S., Rolinski, J., Tabarkiewicz, J., Kolarz, B., Leszczynska-Gorzelak, B., Oleszczuk, J. (2007) Activated T lymphocytes in pre-eclampsia. *Am. J. Reprod. Immunol*, 58, 39-45.

[66] Jonsson, Y., Rubèr, M., Matthiesen, L., Berg, G., Nieminen, K., Sharma, S., et al. (2006) Cytokine mapping of sera from women with preeclampsia and normal pregnancies. *J. Reprod. Immunol*, 70, 83-91.

[67] Borekci, B., Aksoy, H., Demircan, B., Kadanali, S. (2007) Maternal serum interleukin-10, interleukin-2 and interleukin-6 in pre-eclampsia and eclampsia. *Am. J. Reprod. Immunol*, 58, 56-64.

[68] Schiess, B. (2007) Inflammatory response in preeclampsia. *Mol. Aspects Med*, 28, 210-219.

[69] Crocker, I. (2007) Gabor Than Award Lecture 2006: pre-eclampsia and villous trophoblast turnover: perspectives and possibilities. *Placenta,* 28 Suppl A, S4-13.

[70] Saito, S., Shiozaki, A., Nakashima, A., Sakai, M., Sasaki, Y. (2007) The role of the immune system in preeclampsia. *Mol. Aspect. Med.,* 28(2):192-209.

[71] Schiessl, B. (2007) Inflammatory response in preeclampsia. *Mol. Aspect. Med.,* 28(2):210-9.

[72] Sharma, A., Satyam, A., Sharma, J.B. (2007) Leptin, IL-10 and inflammatory markers (TNF-alpha, IL-6 and IL-8) in preeclamptic, normotensive pregnant and healthy non-pregnant women. *Am. J. Reprod. Immunol.,* 58(1):21-30.

[73] Mohaupt, M. (2007) Molecular aspects of preeclampsia. *Mol. Aspect. Med.,* 28(2):169-191.

[74] Luppi, P., DeLoia, J.A. (2006) Monocytes of preeclamptic women spontaneously synthesize pro-inflammatory cytokines. *Clin. Immunol.,* 118(2-3):268-275.

[75] Chen, Q., Viall, C., Kang, Y., Liu, B., Stone, P., Chamley, L. (2009) Antiphospholipid antibodies increase non-apoptotic trophoblast shedding: A contribution to the pathogenesis of pre-eclampsia in affected women? *Placenta,* 30(9):767-773.

[76] Christiansen, O.B., Nielsen, H.S., Kolte, A.M. (2006) Future directions of failed implantation and recurrent miscarriage research. *Reprod. Biomed*, 13, 71-83.

[77] Steele, R.W., Dmowski, W.P., Marmer, D.J. (1984) Immunologic aspects of human endometriosis. *Am. J. Reprod. Immunol.,* 6(1):33-6.

[78] Gui, Y., Zhang, J., Yuan, L., Lessey, B.A. (1999) Regulation of HOXA-10 and its expression in normal and abnormal endometrium. *Mol. Hum. Reprod.,* 5(9), 866-873.

[79] Hastings, J.M., Jackson, K.S., Mavrogianis, A.P.A., Fazleabas, A.T. (2006) The estrogen early response gene FOS is altered in a baboon model of endometriosis. *Biol. Reprod*, 75, 176-182.

[80] Vassiliadis, S., Relakis, K., Papageorgiou, A., Athanassakis, I. (2005) Endometriosis and infertility: a multi-cytokine imbalance versus ovulation, fertilization and early embryo development. *Clin. Dev. Immunol*, 12, 125-129.

In: Immunology in Clinic Practice
Editor: Cagatay Oktenli, pp. 25-46

ISBN 978-1-60876-644-4


*Chapter 3*

# CURRENT PERSPECTIVES ON IMMUNOLOGY AND GERIATRICS

***Uğur Muşabak[1] and Hüseyin Doruk[2]***
1. Department of Immunology,
Gülhane Military Medical Academy, Ankara, Turkey
2. Department of Geriatric Medicine,
Gülhane Military Medical Academy, Ankara, Turkey

## ABSTRACT

Nearly, all organs are affected by ageing process. Functional alterations in central nervous, immune, endocrine and cardiovascular systems take place with age. When age related changes in primary and secondary lymphoid organs are taken into consideration, it seems that the impairment of T cell and B cell functions is inevitable with aging. Immunosenescence may also lead to a state of humoral immune deficiency. Therefore, elderly individuals are more susceptibile to infections than the young individuals. A number of age-related changes in hormonal status may impair the hormone and cytokine network and altere the cytokine milieu of bone marrow. Age-associated alterations in NK cells certainly lead to decline in anti-cancer and anti-viral immunity in elderly individuals. Thus, the age-associated immunodeficiency causes increased susceptibility to cancers, infections, autoimmunity, and cardiovascular disease.

**Keywords:** ageing; aging process; immunosenescence; age-induced changes; elderly; age-associated

## INTRODUCTION

Classically, a balance between inflammatory and anti-inflammatory factors in the host is established in order to elicit an effective immune response to antigens without inflammatory damaging of the tissues [1-9]. Even if different defence mechanisms against pathogens are used by host's both innate and adaptive immune systems, they work in cooperation with each other [8]. The adaptive immune system needs some signals that provide information about the antigen and the type of immune response to be induced. These signals are provided by the innate immune system. On the other hand, adaptive immune cells such as T cell populations have also an important role in determining the nature of the immune response by releasing cytokines [9]. The role of adaptive immune cells in the regulation of immune response might be based on evolutionary relationships between adaptive and innate immunity cells are poorly understood.

Immune system cells are called leukocytes originate from the bone marrow [4]. The precursors of the immune system cells, granulocytes, monocytes, lymphocytes, naturel killer cells mature and differentiate into the specialized cells in the central (primary) lymphoid organs (thymus and bone marrow). While the development of both adaptive and innate immune system in the central lymphoid organs is independent of the antigen, effector and memory cells of adaptive immunity are generated from their naive forms in an antigen dependent manner in the peripheral lymphoid tissues [5]. The cells of innate immunity fight against only the microbes and the responses to these agents occur within a short time frames. Although, the innate immunity is first line and non-specific defence mechanism of the host has restricted specificity by recognizing the pathogen associated molecular paterns (PAMPs) through the the pattern recognition receptors (PRRs). However the specificity of the adaptive immunity has higher than the innate immunity that very fine differences among the antigens can be distinguished by the cells of adaptive immunity [6]. Additionally, discrimination of self from nonself antigens is special to adaptive immune system. Failure of self-nonself discrimination leads to autoimmune diseases. On the other hand, specific memory is an important characteristic of the adaptive immune system and different from the innate immunity. This feature of adaptive immunity ensures the ability to remember the antigen, and to elicit stronger immune responses each time the antigen is encountered. There is also a suppressive function of adaptive immune system on the inflammation by secreting the anti-inflammatory cytokines [7].

## Age Related Changes in Immune System

### 1. Age Related Changes in Immunity

Ageing of immuity is a complex process including the qualitative and quantitative decline of the immune response during aging process. This progressive and irreversibl change in the immunity is also called as immunosenescence [1]. Despite the intensive investigations in the recent years, the pathophysiology of immunosenescence is still not completely understood. On the other hand, there may be large variations among the species and strains. It is widely known that both types of the immune response, innate as well as adaptive, decline with ageing [2]. Impaired immune tolerance is also another age-associated process that increases the susceptibility to autoimmunity [3].

## 2. Age Related Changes in Primary Lymphoid Organs

### *2.1. Bone Marrow*

The pluripotent bone marrow stem cells are capable of differentiation into specialized immune and non-immune cells [10]. The ability of differentiation into multiple cell types is called plasticity or transdifferentiation. Bone marrow stroma contains the cells having many characteristics of stem cells for non-haematopoietic tissues, allowing differentiating into osteoblasts, chondrocytes, adipocytes, and myoblasts [11]. These cells can be defined as mesenchymal due to their differentiation potential into hematopoietic supporting tissues. Hematopoietic compartment of bone marrow developed from stem cells [(Lin-) CD34+] that give rise to myeloid, and lymphoid lineages [12]. However, hematopoietic compartment of bone marrow is replaced by adipose tissue with aging [13]. Stromal cells of bone marrow provide the cytokine milieu required for the development of hematopoietic cell lineages [14]. Despite the fatty changes of bone marrow with age, this process does not influence the number of hematopoietic stem cells [15]. However, the homing and engraftment capability of aged hematopoietic stem cells is substantially declined with age [16].

Many hormones and cytokines from various sources influence the bone marrow morphology and stem cell production. Decreased hormone concentrations and activities including estrogen and testosterone, dehydroepiandrosterone (DHEA) and its sulphate, and the growth hormone (GH)/insulin-like growth factor I systems are determined during normal aging and lead to some phyisiological changes in all of the body's cells and tissues [17,18]. These changes also influence bone marrow and its functions [17]. A study showed that estrogen deficiency causes the increase in bone marrow adipocyte number and size in postmenopausal women [19]. On the other hand, in Bismar et al.'s study, increased bone-resorbing cytokine secretion by human bone marrow cells was found after menopause [20]. It was also shown that estrogen significantly suppresses the production of leukocytes in bone marrow and affects the distribution of polymorphonuclear cells (PMNs) in peripheral blood [21]. Testosterone is other important hormone influences the bone marrow cellularity and functions. Badawi et al. demonsstrated that bone marrow hypoplasia can be improved by testosterone therapy in a patient with panhypopituitarism [22]. In other report, female rats receiving testosterone was found lower fat content in the bone marrow [23]. Similarly, Kim et al. showed that stimulatory effects of androgens on hematopoietic progenitor cells are mostly restricted to mature erythroid progenitors [24]. In this way, while lymphopoiesis is inhibited by DHEA in murine, but myelopoiesis spared [25]. This finding was supported with new studies. Catalina et al. proposed a potential mechanism that increased rate of cellular apoptosis may be resposible for suppression of hematopoiesis by DHEA [26]. In an experimental study in aged rats, hematopoietic bone marrow cells are lower than that of young 3-month-old rats and can be reversed by in vivo treatment with GH [27]. Additionally, age-associated increase in bone marrow adipocytes can also be reversed by GH replacement therapy. These findings support that bone marrow cells are important target for the action of GH [28]. Melatonin is naturally produced in the pineal gland. Melatonin is also synthesized by bone marrow cells that stimulates osteogenic differentiation and inhibits fatty acids-induced adipocytic differentiation of the cells [29]. An experimental study showing melatonin antagonists reverse the effects of melatonin on bone marrow supports these observations.

Therefore, the shift in bone marrow toward fatty changes and osteoporosis development in elderly people have been related to declining melatonin levels with aging.

There are numerous interactions between the neuro-endocrine and immune systems mediated by hormones and cytokines [30]. A number of age-related changes in hormonal status may impair the hormone and cytokine network and altere the cytokine milieu of bone marrow. Disturbed cytokine production may also be, in part, responsible to age-induced changes in bone marrow morphology and stem cell productions [15].

The main cytokines and growth factors that influence the bone marrow, are IL-1, IL-3, IL-5, IL-6, IL-7, IL-11, tumor necrosis factor alpha (TNFα), granulocyte-macrophage colony-stimulating factor (GM-CSF), M-CSF and c-kit ligand [15,31]. All of these cytokines and growth factors play a role in the development of myeloid and lymphoid lineages from hematopoietic stem cells (HSCs). The cytokine balances also change in the ageing process [32]. Increased levels of circulating inflammatory cytokines including TNFα, IL-6 were reporeted in the literature [33]. IL-3 is produced by T cells and stimulates pluripotential hemopoietic stem cell and its derivatives [34], which is also called multi-CSF. In a study, serum levels of IL-3 of active elderly subjects were found similar with young subjects but lower than their sedentary peers. The secretion of IL-7 by aged stromal cells is also decreased with ageing [35]. The other stromal cell derived cytokine is IL-11, which has several biological activities against hematopoietic cells. It was reported that decline in IL-11 expression by stromal cells of bone marrow may play a role in impaired bone formation in the aged population [36]. Additionally, hematopoietic growth factors such as G-CSF, GM-CSF and M-CSF are produced by stromal cells that stimulate the development of inflammatory leukocytes from the progenitor cells of the bone marrow. Diminished production of these hematopoietic growth factors may cause the disordered hematopoiesis in aged population [37].

It is well known that there are many interactions between hormones and cytokines [38]. For example, common intracellular signaling system mediates insulin and some cytokine (IL-2, IL-4, IL-9, interferon (IFN)-γ) action [39]. Thus, simultaneous stimulation of the target cells with both hormones and cytokines can be resulted by antagonistic effect of them on the function of each other. A recent finding showing TNFα impairs activation of signaling elements of the insulin receptor supports this hypothesis [40]. On the other hand, GH, prolactin, and IL-6 also activate same signaling pathways such as signal transducersand activators of transcription (Stat)-5 and Janus kinase (JAK)-Stat [41,42]. When age related hormonal alteration taken into consideration, there may be a strong possibility of changing of hormone-cytokine interactions with ageing.

### *2.2. Thymus*

Mature T cells are generated from bone marrow derived T cell progenitors [43-45] at thymus. There is a sequence of developmental steps in the maturation and differentiation of T cells conducted by cytokines, hormones and thymic microenvironment. Surface expression pattern of T cells is changed in these steps [43,46]. The progenitor cells immigrating into the thymus have CD3-CD4-CD8- surface phenotype. Double negative (DN) cells are further subdivided into four subsets based on their surface expression of CD44 and CD25. DN cells progress to double positive (DP) thymocytes and T cell receptor (TCR) rearrangement takes place at this stage. Double positive T cells undergo positive and negative selection process restricted to major histocompatibility complex (MHC) and 95% of thymocytes die. Meanwhile DP thymocytes decide to become either a CD4+ helper or CD8+ cytotoxic cell. These naive and single positive (SP) cells move out to the perifery and home secondary lymphoid organs.

Thymic T cell output and function progressively declines with ageing due to thymic involution [47,48]. In aged donors, the output of T cells from thymus is measured by decreased TCR excision circle (TREC+) cells [49]. Thymic structure is altered during this process that the thymic epitelial space, in which thymopoesis occurs, attenuates, and perivascular space (adipocytes, stroma) increases with age. However, even into old age, it has been reported that thymus continues to generate new T cells [50]. In spite of continue production of T cells with ageing, naive T cells (CD45RA+) population are depleted in the periphery [51]. The main factors in the development of thymic involution are the changes of the thymic microenvironment and depletion of trophic cytokines, especially IL-7, with ageing [52]. IL-7 plays an important role in thymopoiesis [53]. It was shown that low level IL-7 expression in thymus may decrease thymopoiesis [54]. Additionally, Phillips et al. also reported that the first step of thymopoiesis (DN1-DN2 transition) in aged mice is blocked by decreased intrathymic IL-7 [55]. The other cytokine IFNγ produced by thymocytes induces thymic ephitelial cell activation [56]. On the other hand, TNFα, TGFβ, IL-1β, IL-2, IL-4, IL-6 and IL-10 are also produced in thymus and play a role in T cell development [57-59]. The role of these cytokines on thymopoiesis and the impact of ageing on cytokine network of thymus are still not a fully established up to now [56]. Detailed in vitro and in vivo analysis should be made to explain the effects of ageing on cytokine milieu and T cell development of thymus. In future, these studies may lead to expanded usage of cytokine therapies for induction of thymopoesis in old age. For example, in the thymus of older mice, it was shown that replenish the pool of immature T cells can be achieved through the treatment with IL-7 [60]. However, in other study, IL-7-secreting stromal cell injections into the thymus of aged mice were not found adequate to prevent thymic involution [55]. On the other hand, TNFα has opposite effects (apoptosis/proliferation) on thymocyte production within a broad range of dosages in the presence of IL-7 [61]. In the other study, it was shown that CD8 expression on CD8- thymic subsets including the CD25+CD3-CD4-CD8- pre-T cell subset is induced by adding the combination of TNFα and TGFβ to the thymocyte cultures [62]. Keratinocyte growth factor (KGF), an epithelial cell-specific growth factor, was also examined in aged mice [63]. According to results of Min et al.'s study, it seems that KGF therapy may be clinically useful in improving thymopoiesis and immune function in the elderly. In spite of all these studies, it is still unclear whether systemic or local administration of cytokines in aged humans provides a clinical benefit.

Besides cytokines, some hormones such as leptin and ghrelin play a role in thymopoiesis. Leptin is a hormone that regulates energy intake and energy expenditure [64]. As leptin is also required for normal thymopoiesis, leptin-deficient (ob/ob) mice have severe thymic atrophy [65]. It was shown that leptin administration stimulated thymopoiesis in ob/ob mice. A protecive role of leptin against the setting of inflammation stimuli such as LPS was emphasized in the same study. Despite the conflicting reports on whether circulating leptin levels change during aging, Andrea et al. found that serum leptin concentrations gradually declines during the aging process [66]. However, it was not related to either body mass index (BMI) or other age-related endocrine changes. If the effect of leptin on thymus is considered, leptin administration may be useful for increasing thymopoiesis in aged persons. Dixit et al.

observed that thymocyte counts were significantly increased by leptin infusion in aged but not in young mice [67]. Ghrelin is a protein hormone produced mainly by enteroendocrine cells of that stimulates appetite [67]. This hormone is also produced by immune cells and modulates T cell activation. Additionally, ghrelin expression are found within the thymus and decreased with progressive aging [67]. Therefore, ghrelin and its receptor may have a role in age related thymic involution. Dixit et al.'s study supported this hypothesis that age-associated changes in thymi of 14-month-old mice were significantly improved by infusion of ghrelin [67]. Despite the effect of ghrelin on thymopoiesis is similar to leptin, it is suggested that distinct pathways are used by these hormones for the regulation of thymopoiesis in aged mice. Additionally, it is well known that thymic hormone, thymosin, starts to decline with ageing [68].

## 3. Age Releted Changes in Secondary Lymphoid Organs

Secondary lymphoid organs, also called as peripheral lymphoid organs, consist chiefly of organized lymphoid structures such as the spleen, lymph nodes, and mucosal lympoid tissues. Antigens on professional antigen presenting cells (APCs) are presented firstly to adaptive immune cells within secondary lymphoid organs. The functional arrangement of the cells in secondary lymphoid organs depends on homeostatic growth factors, cytokines and chemokines that attract hematopoietic cells to sites of lymphoid organ and promotes their survival and differentiation [69]. Thus, T cells, B cells and APCs selectively recruit to certain areas in the secondary lymphoid organs. For example, periarteriolar lymphoid sheath (PALS) formed around arterioles is a T cell area in the spleen, which B cell follicles is adjacent to PALS [70]. Antigen presenting cells and macrophages exist in the marginale zone of spleen that is the region at the interface between red pulp and white pulp of the spleen. In other secondary lymphoid organ, lymph node, B cells are recruited in relatively well defined areas known as follicles, surrounded by paracortical T cell area. However, architectural changes also occur in these organs during ageing [15]. Relative spleen weight was observed decreased with age in both C57BL/6 and BALB/c mouse strains [71]. A contrary finding relating to increased splenic weight with age was reported by Cheung et al. [72]. Similar alterations have been observed in lymp nodes [73]. In a study investigating age related changes in the lymph nodes of rats, decrease in the number of germinal centers; loss of cellularity in the cortex; and infiltration of fibroblastic cells in the cortex and the medulla were reported [74]. In other study, age-related decline in the proportion of germinal center B cells from mouse Peyer's patches was reported and found to be accompanied by an accumulation of somatic mutations in their immunoglobulin genes [75]. These age related alterations in secondary lymphoid organs because impaired molecular interactions of the cells such as antigen presentation and antibody production [76].

## 4. Adaptive Immunity in Ageing

Adaptive immune system acts as a second line of defense against invading pathogens. T cells and B cells are major cell types of adaptive immunity. As mentioned before, bone marrow is the main source of both T cells and B cells; and T cells complete their maturation in thymus. When age related changes in primary and secondary lymphoid organs are taken into consideration, it seems that the impairment of T cell and B cell functions is inevitable with aging.

### *4.1. T Cells*

It was shown that naive (virgin) T cell population decreases, memory T cells increase with ageing [77]. These cells are CD4+ and CD8+ T cells that essential to maintain peripheral T cell responses [78,79]. Cytokine production profile of naive T cells also change with ageing. A T helper (Th) 1 type cytokine, IL-2 and Th2 type cytokines, IL-4 and IL-5 produced by memory cells derived from older naive cells are less than those of memory cells generated from younger naive cells [80,81]. The expression of CD40L on the CD4+ T cells diminishes with ageing due to decreased IL-2 secretion. The defective interaction between CD40L and CD40 results in alteration in the interactions of T cells and B cells. This alteration in aged T cell-B cell interaction impairs the antibody production. The other consequence, delayed cytotoxic T cell response to viral agents, is also based on age related alterations of CD4+ T cells [82]. The defect in aged cytotoxic T cells has less capability of binding to their target [83]. However, destroying effect of cytotoxic T cells does not change with ageing.

Declined proliferative response to mitogens is another age related qualitative alteration of T cells [84]. This defect based on impaired regulation between stimulatory and inhibitory genes of DNA replication causes to decrese in T cells entering active replication phase [85]. The p53 gene plays a regulatory role in apoptosis and its expression decreases in active T cells form in aged donors [86].

Regulatory T cells (Treg) have suppressive effect on immune response that also plays an essential role in the maintenance of immunological tolerance [87]. There are two major subsets of Treg cells (CD4+CD25+) including the natural Treg cells and the adaptive Treg cells. Naturally occurring CD4+CD25+ Treg cells arise in thymus and constitute 5-10% of the total peripheral CD4+ T cells [88]. Several activation markers, the glucocorticoid-induced TNF receptor-related protein (GITR), OX40 (CD134), cytotoxic T lymphocyte associated antigen 4 (CTLA-4 or CD152), and L-selectin are also constitutively expressed in these cells. Neither CD25 nor the other activation molecules are reliable markers for the identification of Tregs. However, in recent studies, the transcription factor forkhead box P3 (FOXP3) was identified as a more spesific intracellular marker of naturally occurring Treg cells [89]. Adaptive Treg cells seem non-regulatory CD4+ T-cells that arise in the periphery upon encountering antigen. The CD25 molecule expression in adaptive Treg cells is upregulated during infectious and inflammatory conditions.

One of the the proposed suppression mechanisms of Treg is direct cell-cell contact dependent mechanism that mediated by CTLA-4 on both effector T cells and APCs. The production of immunosuppressive cytokines (IL-10, TGF-β) by Tregs is other mechanism that suppresses DC maturation by making DCs tolerogenic. The last mechanism is the killing ability of Tregs on effector T cells by expression of perforin and granzyme [87].

The results of studies investigating age associated quantitative and qualitative changes in Treg cell are contraversial. Greg et al. have shown that the number of peripheral blood CD4+CD25+ Treg cells in elderly donors' increases with ageing without alteration their regulatory function [90]. Similar results were found in Nishioka et al.'s study that CD4+CD25+ Treg cells in aged mice are functionally comparable to those in young mice, although slightly increased in number [91]. Tsaknaridis et al. also suggested that suppressive activity of human CD4+CD25+ T cells does not change with age. [92]. Accordingly, it may be reasonably speculated that impaired adaptive immune response are related to the increasing CD4+CD25+ Treg cells numbers and correlated with age. Therfore, an imbalance of Treg homeostasis may predispose elderly individuals to infections, immune-mediated diseases, or cancers [93]. However, further studies are needed to clarify these controversies.

### *4.2. B Cells*

According to results of comperative analysis, the alterations in B cell population may be associated or not with ageing. Ligthart et al. already reported that the number of B cells in the peripheral bloods of elderly individuals was slightly decreased compared to younger individuals [94]. The other study showing to be declined capability of the bone marrow to generate new B cells in aging seems to support Ligthart et al.'s study [95]. During ageing, alterations in B-cell development include both a skewing of V-gene utilization and a decline in the generation of various developmental B-cell subsets [96]. In a new study using aged mice, it was reported that while moderate loss of late-stage pre-B cells resulted with decrease in proliferation to IL-7 and decrease in the frequency of pro-B cells which increased response upon IL-7 stimulation, a severe loss of pre-B cells resulted in a reduced pro-B cell pool which retained normal activation and proliferative responses to IL-7 [97]. Additionally, the increased susceptibility to apoptosis in B cell precursors from aged mice with severe alterations in B lymphopoiesis compared to both aged mice with moderate B cell precursor loss and young individuals was found in Van der Put et al's study [97]. Therefore, it was proposed that refractory B cell precursors initially accumulated in aged mice which are poorly responsive to IL-7 may be eliminated via apoptosis; but, the remaining limited pool of B cell precursors retains the capacity to respond to IL-7 stimulation. As mentioned before, age related changes in B cell population also occur in B cell rich areas of peripheral lymphoid tissues such as spleen, lymp nodes and peyer plaques.

In the literature, there are several studies demonstrating functional alterations of peripheral B cells in elderly individuals [98]. In a study, splenic B lymphocytes from aged mice were found to exhibit lower level of apoptosis induced by B-cell antigen receptor (BCR) ligation, but intact susceptibility to anti-Fas induced apoptosis in vitro [99]. However, an increased proliferative response and similar level of activation markers expression upon BCR stimulation are presented by aged B cells compared to those of B cells from young mice. Age-related T cell alterations lead to decrease in T dependent B cell functions [100]. It is well known that T lymphocytes are more severely affected than B cells and T cell dependent antibody production decreases with ageing [101]. On the other hand, B cell repertoire which is specific for different antigens changes with age [102]. The proposed mechanism for this change are age associated impairment in the production of a diverse population of naive B cells in the bone marrow and the decreased diversification of B cells in the germinal center where affinity maturation and isotype switching takes place. Thus, age related changes in B cells cause the alterations of the antibody response including shifts in antibody specificities from foreign to autoantigens, in antibody affinities from high to low, in antibody isotypes from IgG to IgM, and in the antibody idiotypic repertoire [103,104]. Age related T cell impairments may play an important role in this humoral immune dysregulation [104]. A study supports that humoral immune dysregulation exists in old mice and the immunization with foreing antigens causes polyreactive IgM response which react with autoantigens [105]. In other study, it was shown that specific antibody response against specific antigens declines in aged individuals. In Kishimoto et al.'s study, age associated decline in proportions of B-cell precursors and specific Th cells involved in the IgG anti-tetanus toxoid antibody production was found in humans [106]. Additionally, antibody responses to different doses of influenza vaccine were found different in elderly in comparison to young individuals [107]. In Remarque et al.'s study, the IgM, IgG3 and IgA1 responses at a 10 micrograms dose of influenza vaccine were found similar in both elderly and young individuls, whereas the IgG, IgG1 and haemagglutination inhibition (HI) responses were found two fold lower in the elderly individuals compared to young subjects. In other study, it was demonstrated that there were increased occurrence of CD8(+)CD28(-) T cell clonal expansions in elderly donors who fail to produce antibody against influenza vaccination [108]. It seems likely that elderly individuals are more susceptibile to infections than the young individuals. Thus, immunosenescence may also lead to a state of humoral immune deficiency.

### *4.3. Dendritic Cells*

Dendritic cells (DCs) are a heterogeneous group of cells that derived from myeloid or lymphid progenitor cells [109]. These subtypes are called as myeloid DCs (MDCs) and plasmacytoid DCs (PDCs), respectively [110]. They are found in most tissues and organs of the body, especially abundant in those that are interfaces between the external and internal environments such as integumentary and gastrointestinal systems.

Dendritic cells are known as professional APCs, with a strong capacity for initiating naive T-cell response [111]. It is well known that DCs bridge the innate and acquired immune systems. The antigens in peripheral tissues are captured by DCs and carried to secondary lymphoid tissues via the lymphatic vessels. These antigens are presented to naive lymphocytes in secondary lymphoid tissues [112,113]. The mechanisms of antigen capture in DC are receptor mediated endocytosis, macropinocytosis, and phagocytosis [114]. The shift in Th1/Th2 immune responses is directed by DC cytokines such as IL-12 and IL-18. Therefore, DCs play a central role in initiating the primary immune response. On the other hand, IL-10, a key cytokine, that can suppress Th1 type immunity and maturation of DC subsets.

Recent investigations have focused on DCs and age associated alterations within DC function. Fujihashi et al. reported that decreased DCs in Peyer's patches of elderly individuals partially impair mucosal immune regulation [115]. Thus, age associated mucosal dysregulation breaks down the induction of either sIgA immunity or oral tolerance. In other study, the numbers of langerhans cells (LCs) were found decreased in aged skin [116]. Zavala et al. was found altered expression levels of CD1a on LCs in gingival epithelium from elderly individuals [117]. It was also shown that DCs and T cells number increase in brain areas where substantial histopathological changes and a volumetric decrease are observed in aging mice [118].

Besides the phenotypic changes of DCs with ageing, functional alterations are also observed in aged DCs. Agrawal et al reported that both receptor-dependent and receptor-independent antigen capture mechanisms are decreased in monocyte derived DCs from aged humans [119]. Additionally, the clearence of apoptotic cells by phagocytes was found to be defective in elderly individuals. It is well known that apoptotic cells are a potential source of autoantigens and, therefore, their inefficient elimination lead to necrotic cell death. While the apoptotic cells inhibit the DCs, necrotic cells stimulate the DCs and proinflammatory cytokine production [120]. Thus released autoantigens in elderly individuals are captured by DCs and presented to adaptive immune system resulting chronic inflammation and autoimmunity. The pro-inflammatory cytokines (i.e. TNFα, IL-6) are secreted at high levels upon TLR stimulation in elderly subjects [121]. On the other hand, this declined phagocytic capability of DCs increases susceptibility to infections.

As mentioned before, Th1 or Th2 development is induced by DCs, and this regulation are impaired with ageing. According to a new study, a Th1 type immune response predominates in healthy individuals and a Th2 response predominates in elderly individuals [122]. This finding may be reasonably explained by increased IL-10 production in elderly individuals [123]. On the other hand, costimulatory molecule expression and cytokine and chemokine secretion were found to be defective in aged APCs that lead to poor T cell clonal expansion and function [124]. Similar results was reported in a previous study that DC from aged senescence-accelerated mouse (SAMP1) mice showed less stimulatory activity than those of age-matched BALB/c or young SAMP1 mice [125].

## 5. Innate Immunity in Ageing

The innate immune system acts as the first line of defense against invading pathogens. Cellular components of the innate immune system, mainly macrophages, natural killer (NK) cells and PMNs. Ageing also affects this system and lead to increased susceptibility to infections and cancers.

### *5.1. Macrophages*

Macrophages develop from the myeloid lineage in bone marrow under the influence of various growth factors including GM-CSF, M-CSF. It was reported that macrophage precursors decline in bone marrow with ageing [126]. Tissue forms of macrophages have specialized properties such as LCs in skin, kupffer cells in liver and microglia in brain. Langerhans cells and their functions were found to be decreased in elderly subjects [127].

Macrophages and DCs have a set of transmembrane receptors that recognize different types of pathogen-associated molecular patterns (PAMPs). These transmembrane molecules are called as pattern recognition receptors (PRRs). PAMPs are small molecular structures on microbes, and microbial products. Toll-like receptors are a subtype of PRRs, and TLR-PAMP interaction in macrophages induces the release of proinflammatory cytokines such as TNFα and IL-6 [128,129]. Thus, invading pathogens are eliminated by triggered inflammatory response. Impaired TLR expression in aged macrophage may be partly responsible for increased susceptibility to bacterial, fungal, and viral infections in elderly individuals. The defect in TLR signalling pathway of aged macrophages leads to decrease in cytokine production of macrophages [129].

The effect of ageing on phagocytic function of macrophages is not clear. However, several study using animal models shown that there are phagocytic dysfunction and impaired oxidative burst activity in aged animals [128,129]. It was proposed that fagocytic dysfunction in aged animals depends on deficits in phacytosis promoting receptor expression (e.g. mannose receptor, scavenger receptor, CD14, CD36) and their signalling mechanism. Abnormal response to chemotactic stimuli is the other dysfunction of aged macrophages

[128,129]. Fietta et al. proposed that impaired macrophage chemotaxis against compleman derived factors leads to delayed pathogen clearence in elderly individuals [130]. Ortega et al. has presented some confilicting results regarding the macrophage functions [131]. In their study, the adherence capacity of peritoneal macrophages was found greater in adult (24 weeks) and old mice (72 weeks) than in young animals (12 weeks). However, the chemotaxis of macrophages was found higher in cells from young mice than in those from adult mice, and chemotactic activity was again found increased in macrophages from mature (48 weeks) and old animals. In the same study, similar patterns were also observed in phagocytic activity and anion superoxide production of aged macrophages.

### *5.2. Polymorphonuclear Leukocytes*

Polymorphonuclear leukocytes (PMNs) play an important role in the defense against infectious agents. The main functions of PMNs are phagocytosis, oxidative burst, and intracellular killing of microbes. [132]. They have a short-life span and die by spontaneous apoptosis. They are derived from myeloid lineage and released from bone marrow to systemic circulation [133]. Colony stimulating factors such as G-CSF and GM-CSF stimulate PMN production and survival [134]. Infections and inflammations shorten the transit time of PMN in the marrow by inflammatory cytokines such as IL-1, IL-6, IL-8, and TNFα [135-137].

Ageing also affects qualitative and quantitative characteristics of PMNs. In an erlier report, it was mentioned that there is a functional granulocytopenia in the elderly individuals in spite of normal numbers of PMNs being present [138]. In other report, it was also underlined that the number of circulating neutrophils, but not their phagocytic ability and intracellular killing capacity, remains unaltered in the elderly compared with young [139]. Similar results were also reported by Wenisch et al. [140]. In Gocer et al.'s study, despite the intracellular killing activity of PMNs was found decreased in elderly patients; phagocytic activitiy was found intact [141]. The study presented by Angelis et al. seems to be different on account of its results. Accorrding to their study, age is not associated with an alteration in PMN number or activity in the absence of bacterial infection. Additionally, infection in both young and elderly produces a significant increase in neutrophil number and chemiluminescence activity [142].

On the other hand, age-related changes in cell adhesion molecule (CAM) expression on PMNs surfaces could be partially responsible for immune dysfunctions during ageing [143]. It is well known that CAMs involved in the migration of PMNs to inflamed tissues. Several studies shown that CAM mediated chemotaxis of PMNs are defective in old age. In a study, the percentage of granulocytes and monocytes expressing CD62L was found decreased in the elderly, whereas its density expression was found unchanged on both cell type [143]. According to this study results, the authors suggested that the increased proportion of CD62L negative granulocytes in the elderly leads to impairment in cell adhesion and this phenomenon likely contributes to the increased susceptibility to acute infections of elderly people.

### *5.3. Natural Killer Cells*

Natural killer cells belong to the innate immune system, and play an important role in kiiling tumor cells, and virally infected cells [144]. They do not need activation for their killing functions. Despite the phenotype of NK is closely similar to T cells, NK cells do not express the TCR-CD3 complex. Lymphokine activated killer (LAK) cells are generated by incubation of NK cells with recombinant IL-2 and also found in peripheral blood [145]. The cytotoxic activities NK and LAK cells are different from each other [146]. The other subtype, natural killer T (NKT) cell, is a unique subset of T cells that this cell recognizes the non-polymorphic CD1d molecule [147]. The features of NKT cells share properties of both T cells and NK cells.

Age-associated changes in NK cells have also been demonstrated [148]. While a significant expansion in the percentage of NK cells showing a mature phenotype are observed in elderly donors, NK cell cytotoxicity decreases in aging [148,149]. Speculatively, the increase in the number and percentage of NK cells with age could be a compensatory mechanism to overwhelm the reduced cytolytic activity of NK cells [150]. Similar findings were reported by McNerlan et al. that there has been a significant increase in both the absolute counts and the proportions of CD3-CD(16+56)+ (NK cells) and CD3+CD(16+56)+ (NKT cells) with age, and NK cell subsets. In the same study, soluble IL-2 receptor levels were also found to increase significantly with age and correlated with certain NK cell subsets [151]. While, CD56bright NK cells are the major cytokine producing subset, CD56dim NK cells exhibit greater cytotoxic activity. There are also contrary results in the literature with respect to age associated qualitative and quantitative changes in NK cells. For example, in a study, the number of NK (CD56+CD3-) cells within peripheral blood was found stabil with ageing [152]. In Chidrawar et al.'s study, the number of CD56dim NK cells within peripheral blood in elderly individuals was not different from young adults, whereas the absolute number of CD56bright NK cells was found declined in aged individuals compared to young adults. These alterations in NK cells certainly lead to decline in anti-cancer and anti-viral immunity in elderly individuals [153,154].

## Conclusion

Immunosenescence can be shortly defined as age associated deterioration in immune functions. Age-associated changes in immunity are observed not only in adaptive immunity, but also in innate immunity. Poor quality of immune response in elderly individuals increases the susceptibility of cancers, infectious disease and autoimmune diseases. It seems that the accumulated data from the studies focusing on immunology of ageing until now will possibly lead to solve complex immunosenescence mechanisms and discover a new therapy models for reversal of ageing changes in immunity.

## References

[1] Cambier, J. (2005). Immunosenescence: a problem of lymphopoiesis, homeostasis, microenvironment, and signaling. *Immunol. Rev*, 205, 5-6.

[2] Kumar, R., Burns, E.A. (2008). Age-related decline in immunity: implications for vaccine responsiveness. *Expert Rev. Vaccines*, 7, 467-473.

[3] Fülöp, T. Jr., Larbi, A., Dupuis, G., Pawelec, G. (2003) Ageing, autoimmunity and arthritis: Perturbations of TCR signal transduction pathways with ageing - a biochemical paradigm for the ageing immune system. *Arthritis Res. Ther*, 5, 290-302.

[4] Obinata, M., Okuyama, R., Matsuda, K.I., Koguma, M., Yanai, N. (1998) Regulation of myeloid and lymphoid development of hematopoietic stem cells by bone marrow stromal cells. *Leuk. Lymphoma*, 29, 61-69.

[5] Boes, M., Ploegh, H.L. (2004) Translating cell biology in vitro to immunity in vivo. *Nature*, 8, 430, 264-271.

[6] Vivier, E., Malissen, B. (2005) Innate and adaptive immunity: specificities and signaling hierarchies revisited. *Nat. Immunol*, 6, 17-21.

[7] Opal, S.M., DePalo, V.A. (2000) Anti-inflammatory cytokines.*Chest*, 117, 1162-1172.

[8] Palm, N.W., Medzhitov, R. (2007) Not so fast: adaptive suppression of innate immunity. *Nat. Med*, 13, 1142-1144.

[9] Pulendran, B. (2004) Modulating TH1/TH2 responses with microbes, dendritic cells, and pathogen recognition receptors. *Immunol. Res*, 29, 187-196.

[10] [http://stemcells.nih.gov/info/basics/basics4.asp].

[11] Prockop, D.J. (1997) Marrow stromal cells as stem cells for nonhematopoietic tissues. *Science*, 276, 71-74.

[12] Kohn, D.B., Bauer, G., Rice, C.R., Rothschild, J.C., Carbonaro, D.A., Valdez, P., et al., (1999) A clinical trial of retroviral-mediated transfer of a rev-responsive element decoy gene into CD34(+) cells from the bone marrow of human immunodeficiency virus-1-infected children. *Blood*, 1, 94, 368-371.

[13] Justesen, J., Stenderup, K., Ebbesen, E.N., Mosekilde, L., Steiniche T., Kasem, M. (2001) Adipocyte tissue volume in bone marrow is increased with aging and in patients with osteoporosis. *Biogerontology*, 2, 165-171.

[14] Jensen, B.A., Leeman, R.J., Schlezinger, J.J., Sherr, D.H. (2003) Aryl hydrocarbon receptor (AhR) agonists suppress interleukin-6 expression by bone marrow stromal cells: an immunotoxicology study. *Environ. Health*, 16, 2, 16.

[15] Gruver, A.L., Hudson, L.L., Sempowski, G.D. (2007) Immunosenescence of ageing. *J. Pathol*, 211, 144-156.

[16] Liang, Y., Van Zant, G., Szilvassy, S.J. (2005) Effects of aging on the homing and engraftment of murine hematopoietic stem and progenitor cells. *Blood*, 106, 1479-1487.

[17] Thorner, M.O. (2009) Statement by the Growth Hormone Research Society on the GH/IGF-I Axis in Extending Health Span. *J. Gerontol. A Biol. Sci. Med. Sci*, Jul 8. [Epub ahead of print]

[18] Cappola, A.R., Xue, Q.L., Fried, L.P. (2009) Multiple hormonal deficiencies in anabolic hormones are found in frail older women: the Women's Health and Aging studies. *J. Gerontol. A Biol. Sci. Med. Sci*, 64, 243-248.

[19] Syed, F.A., Oursler, M.J., Hefferanm, T.E., Peterson, J.M., Riggs, B.L., Khosla, S. (2008) Effects of estrogen therapy on bone marrow adipocytes in postmenopausal osteoporotic women. *Osteoporos Int*, 19, 1323-1330.

[20] Bismar, H., Diel, I., Ziegler, R., Pfeilschifter, J. (1995) Increased cytokine secretion by human bone marrow cells after menopause or discontinuation of estrogen replacement. *J. Clin. Endocrinol. Metab*, 80, 3351-3355.

[21] Josefsson, E., Tarkowski, A., Carlsten, H. (1992) Anti-inflammatory properties of estrogen. I. In vivo suppression of leukocyte production in bone marrow and redistribution of peripheral blood neutrophils. *Cell Immunol*, 142, 67-78.
[22] Badawi, M.A., Salih, F., Al-Humaidi, A.A., El Khalifa, M.Y., Elhadd, T.A. (2008) Bone marrow hypoplasia responsive to testosterone therapy in a patient with panhypopituitarism: need for adherence to androgen replacement. *Endocr. Pract*, 4, 229-232.
[23] Tamura, N., Kurabayashi, T., Nagata, H., Matsushita, H., Yahata, T., Tanaka, K. (2005) Effects of testosterone on cancellous bone, marrow adipocytes, and ovarian phenotype in a young female rat model of polycystic ovary syndrome. *Fertil Steril*, 84, 2, 1277-1284.
[24] Kim, S.W., Hwang, J.H., Cheon, J.M., Park, N.S., Park, S.E., Park, S.J., et al., (2005) Direct and indirect effects of androgens on survival of hematopoietic progenitor cells in vitro. *J. Korean Med. Sci*, 20, 409-416.
[25] Risdon, G., Kumar, V., Bennett M. (1991) Differential effects of dehydroepiandrosterone (DHEA) on murine lymphopoiesis and myelopoiesis. *Exp. Hematol*, 19, 128-131.
[26] Catalina, F., Milewich, L., Kumar, V., Bennett, M. (2003) Dietary dehydroepiandrosterone inhibits bone marrow and leukemia cell transplants: role of food restriction. *Exp. Biol. Med*, 228, 1303-1320.
[27] French, R.A., Broussard, S.R., Meier, W.A., Minshall, C., Arkins, S., Zachary, J.F., Dantzer, R., Kelley, K.W. (2002) Age-associated loss of bone marrow hematopoietic cells is reversed by GH and accompanies thymic reconstitution. *Endocrinology*, 143, 690-699.
[28] Welniak, L.A., Tian, Z.G., Sun, R., Keller, J.R., Richards, S., Ruscetti, F.W., Murphy, W.J. (2000) Effects of growth hormone and prolactin on hematopoiesis. *Leuk. Lymphoma*, 38, 435-445.
[29] Sanchez-Hidalgo, M., Lu, Z., Tan, D.X., Maldonado, M.D., Reiter, R.J., Gregerman, R.I. (2007) Melatonin inhibits fatty acid-induced triglyceride accumulation in ROS17/2.8 cells: implications for osteoblast differentiation and osteoporosis. *Am. J. Physiol. Regul. Integr. Comp. Physiol*, 292, R2208-15.
[30] Mazzoccoli, G., Correra, M., Bianco, G., De Cata, A., Balzanelli, M., Giuliani, A., Tarquini, R. (1997) Age-related changes of neuro-endocrine-immune interactions in healthy humans. *J. Biol. Regul. Homeost Agents*, 11, 143-147.
[31] Abbas, A.K., Lichtman, A.H. (2003) Cellular and Molecular Immunology, Philadelphia. Saunders, Chapter 11.
[32] Bruunsgaard, H., Pedersen, M., Pedersen, B.K. (2001) Aging and proinflammatory cytokines. *Curr. Opin. Hematol*, 8, 131-136.
[33] Dobbs, R.J., Charlett, A., Purkiss, A.G. (1999) Association of circulating TNF-alpha and IL-6 with ageing and Parkinsonism. *Acta Neurol. Scand*, 100, 34-41.
[34] Arai, M.H., Duarte, A.J., Natale, V.M. (2006) The effects of long-term endurance training on the immune and endocrine systems of elderly men: the role of cytokines and anabolic hormones. *Immun. Ageing*, 25, 3, 9.
[35] Miller, J.P., Izon, D., DeMuth, W., Gerstein, R., Bhandoola, A., Alman, D. (2002) The earliest step in B lineage differentiation from common lymphoid progenitors is critically dependent upon interleukin 7. *J. Exp. Med*, 2, 196, 705-711.

[36] Tohjima, E., Inoue, D., Yamamoto, N., Kido, S., Ito, Y., Kato, S., et al., (2003) Decreased AP-1 activity and interleukin-11 expression by bone marrow stromal cells may be associated with impaired bone formation in aged mice. *J. Bone Miner. Res*, 18, 1461-1470.
[37] Buchanan, J.P., Peters, C.A., Rasmussen, C.J., Rothstein, G. (1996) Impaired expression of hematopoietic growth factors: a candidate mechanism for the hematopoietic defect of aging. *Exp. Gerontol*, 31, 135-144.
[38] Broussard, S.R., McCusker, R.H., Novakofski, J.E., Strle, K., Shen, W.H., Johnson, R.W., et al., (2003) Cytokine-hormone interactions: tumor necrosis factor alpha impairs biologic activity and downstream activation signals of the insulin-like growth factor I receptor in myoblasts. *Endocrinology*, 144, 2988-2996.
[39] White, M.F., Yenush, L. (1998) The IRS-signaling system: a network of docking proteins that mediate insulin and cytokine action. *Curr. Top Microbiol. Immunol*, 228, 179-208.
[40] Hirosumi, J., Tuncman, G., Chang, L., Gorgun, C.Z., Uysal, K.T., Maeda, K., et al., (2002) A central role for JNK in obesity and insulin resistance. *Nature*, 420, 333-336.
[41] Groner, B., and Gouilleux, F. (1995) Prolactin-mediated gene activation in mammary epithelial cells. *Curr. Opin. Genet Dev*, 5, 587-594.
[42] Kelly, P.A., Bachelot, A., Kedzia, C., Hennighausen, L., Ormandy, C.J., Kopchick, J.J., Binart, N. (2002) The role of prolactin and growth hormone in mammary gland development. *Mol. Cell Endocrinol*, 197, 127-131.
[43] Kaye, J. (2000) Regulation of T cell development in the thymus. *Immunol. Res*, 21, 71-81.
[44] Page, D.M., Kane, L.P., Allison, J.P., Hedrick, SM. (1993) Two signals are required for negative selection of CD4+CD8+ thymocytes. *J. Immunol*, 15, 151, 1868-1680.
[45] Punt, J.A., Suzuki, H., Granger, L.G., Sharrow, S.O., Singer, A. (1996) Lineage commitment in the thymus: only the most differentiated (TCRhibcl-2hi) subset of CD4+CD8+ thymocytes has selectively terminated CD4 or CD8 synthesis. *J. Exp. Med*, 184, 2091-2099.
[46] Haynes, B.F. (1990) Human thymic epithelium and T cell development: current issues and future directions. *Thymus*, 16, 143-157.
[47] George, A.J., Ritter, M.A. (1996) Thymic involution with ageing: obsolescence or good housekeeping? *Immunol. Today*, 17, 267-272.
[48] Hazenberg, M.D., Borghans, J.A, de Boer, R.J., Miedema, F. (2003) Thymic output: a bad TREC record. *Nat. Immunol*, 4, 97-99.
[49] Haynes, B.F., Markert, M.L., Sempowski, G.D., Patel, D.D., Hale, L.P. (2000) The role of the thymus in immune reconstitution in aging, bone marrow transplantation, and HIV-1 infection. *Annu. Rev. Immunol*, 18, 529-560.
[50] Hakim, F.T., Memon, S.A., Cepeda, R., Jones, E.C., Chow, C.K., Kasten-Sportes, C., et al., (2005) Age-dependent incidence, time course, and consequences of thymic renewal in adults. *J. Clin. Invest*, 115, 930-939.
[51] Cicin-Sain, L., Messaoudi, I., Park, B., Currier, N., Planer, S., Fischer, M., et al., (2007) Dramatic increase in naive T cell turnover is linked to loss of naive T cells from old primates. *Proc. Natl. Acad. Sci*, 11, 104, 19960-5.

[52] Plum, J., De Smedt, M., Leclercq, G., Verhasselt, B., Vandekerckhove, B. (1996) Interleukin-7 is a critical growth factor in early human T-cell development. *Blood*, 88, 4239-4245.

[53] Okamoto, Y., Douek, D.C., McFarland, R.D., Koup, R.A. (2002) IL-7, the thymus, and naïve T cells. *Adv. Exp. Med. Biol*, 512, 81-90.

[54] Andrew, D., Aspinall, R. (2002) Age-associated thymic atrophy is linked to a decline in IL-7 production. *Exp. Gerontol*, 37, 455-463.

[55] Phillips, J.A., Brondstetter, T.I., English, C.A., Lee, H.E., Virts, E.L., Thoman, M.L. (2004) IL-7 gene therapy in aging restores early thymopoiesis without reversing involution. *J. Immunol*, 15, 173, 4867-4874.

[56] Yarilin, A.A., Belyakov, IM. (2004) Cytokines in the thymus: production and biological effects. *Curr. Med. Chem*, 11, 447-464.

[57] Deman, J., Van Meurs, M., Claassen, E., Humblet, C., Boniver, J., Defresne, M.P. (1996) In vivo expression of interleukin-1 beta (IL-1 beta), IL-2, IL-4, IL-6, tumour necrosis factor-alpha and interferon-gamma in the fetal murine thymus. *Immunology*, 89, 152-157.

[58] Karpuzoglu-Sahin, E., Zhi-Jun, Y., Lengi, A., Sriranganathan, N., Ansar Ahmed, S. (2001), Effects of long-term estrogen treatment on IFN-gamma, IL-2 and IL-4 gene expression and protein synthesis in spleen and thymus of normal C57BL/6 mice. *Cytokine*, 21, 14, 208-217.

[59] Plum, J., De Smedt, M., Leclercq, G., Vandekerckhove, B. (1995) Influence of TGF-beta on murine thymocyte development in fetal thymus organ culture. *J. Immunol*, 154, 5789-5798.

[60] Andrew, D., Aspinall, R. (2001) Il-7 and not stem cell factor reverses both the increase in apoptosis and the decline in thymopoiesis seen in aged mice. *J. Immunol*, 166, 1524-1530.

[61] Baseta, JG., Stutman, O. (2000) TNF regulates thymocyte production by apoptosis and proliferation of the triple negative (CD3-CD4-CD8-) subset. *J. Immunol*, 165, 5621-5630.

[62] Suda, T., Zlotnik, A. (1992) In vitro induction of CD8 expression on thymic pre-T cells. I. Transforming growth factor-beta and tumor necrosis factor-alpha induce CD8 expression on CD8- thymic subsets including the CD25+CD3-CD4-CD8- pre-T cell subset. *J. Immunol*, 148, 1737-1745.

[63] Min, D., Panoskaltsis-Mortari, A., Kuro-O, M., Holländer, G.A., Blazar, B.R., Weinberg, K.I. (2007) Sustained thymopoiesis and improvement in functional immunity induced by exogenous KGF administration in murine models of aging. *Blood*, 109, 2529-2537.

[64] Blüher, S., Mantzoros, C.S. (2004) The role of leptin in regulating neuroendocrine function in humans. *J. Nutr*, 134, 2469S-2474S.

[65] Hick, R.W., Gruver, A.L., Ventevogel, M.S., Haynes, B.F., Sempowski, G.D. (2006) Leptin selectively augments thymopoiesis in leptin deficiency and lipopolysaccharide-induced thymic atrophy. *J. Immunol*, 177, 169-176.

[66] Isidori, A.M., Strollo, F., Morè, M., Caprio, M., Aversa, A., Moretti, C., et al., (2000) Leptin and aging: correlation with endocrine changes in male and female healthy adult populations of different body weights. *J. Clin. Endocrinol. Metab*, 85, 1954-1962.

[67] Dixit, V.D., Yang, H., Sun, Y., Weeraratna, A.T., Youm, Y.H., SmithR.G., Taub, D.D. (2007) Ghrelin promotes thymopoiesis during aging. *J. Clin. Invest*, 117, 2778-2790.

[68] Song, L., Kim, Y.H., Chopra, R.K., Proust, J.J., Nagel, J.E., Nordin, A.A., Adler, W.H. (1993) Age-related effects in T cell activation and proliferation. *Exp. Gerontol*, 28, 313-321.

[69] Randall, T.D., Carragher, D.M., Rangel-Moreno, J. (2008) Development of secondary lymphoid organs. *Annu. Rev. Immunol*, 26, 627-650.

[70] Cook, M.C., Basten, A., Fazekas de St Groth, B. (1997) Outer periarteriolar lymphoid sheath arrest and subsequent differentiation of both naive and tolerant immunoglobulin transgenic B cells is determined by B cell receptor occupancy. *J. Exp. Med*, 29, 186, 631-643.

[71] Pinchuk, L.M., Filipov, N.M. (2008) Endothelial nitric oxide synthase gene polymorphisms and cardiovascular damage in hypertensive subjects: an Italian case-control study. *Immun. Ageing*, 11, 5, 4.

[72] Cheung, H.T., Nadakavukaren, M.J. (1983) Age-dependent changes in the cellularity and ultrastructure of the spleen of Fischer F344 rats. *Mech. Ageing Dev*, 22, 23-33.

[73] Hoffman-Goetz L, Thorne R, Simpson JA, Arumugam Y (1989) Exercise stress alters murine lymphocyte subset distribution in spleen, lymph nodes and thymus. *Clin. Exp. Immunol*, 76, 307-310.

[74] Pahlavani, M.A., Richardson, A., Cheung, H.T. (1987) Age-dependent changes of the mesenteric lymph node of Fischer F344 rats: morphological and histometric analysis. *Mech. Ageing Dev*, 39, 137-146.

[75] González-Fernández, A., Gilmore, D., Milstein, C. (1994) Age-related decrease in the proportion of germinal center B cells from mouse Peyer's patches is accompanied by an accumulation of somatic mutations in their immunoglobulin genes. *Eur. J. Immunol*, 24, 2918-2921.

[76] Szakal, A.K., Aydar, Y., Balogh, P., Tew, J.G. (2002) Molecular interactions of FDCs with B cells in aging. *Semin. Immunol*, 14, 267-274.

[77] Pahlavani, M.A., Vargas, D.M. (2000) Influence of aging and caloric restriction on activation of Ras/MAPK, calcineurin, and CaMK-IV activities in rat T cells. *Proc. Soc. Exp. Biol. Med*, 223, 163-169.

[78] Kudlacek, S., Jahandideh-Kazempour, S., Graninger, W., Willvonseder, R., Pietschmann, P. (1995) Differential expression of various T cell surface markers in young and elderly subjects. *Immunobiology*, 192, 198-204.

[79] Jackola, D.R., Ruger, J.K., Miller, R.A. (1994) Age-associated changes in human T cell phenotype and function. *Aging (Milano)*, 6, 25-34.

[80] Haynes, L., Eaton, S.M., Burns, E.M., Randall, T.D., Swain, S.L. (2005) Newly generated CD4 T cells in aged animals do not exhibit age-related defects in response to antigen. *J. Exp. Med*, 201, 845-851.

[81] Haynes, L., Eaton, S.M., Burns, E.M., Randall, T.D., Swain, S.L. (2003) CD4 T cell memory derived from young naive cells functions well into old age, but memory generated from aged naive cells functions poorly. *Proc. Natl. Acad. Sci*, 100, 15053-8.

[82] Vissinga, C., Nagelkerken, L., Zijlstra, J., Hertogh-Huijbregts, A., Boersma, W., Rozing, J. (1990) A decreased functional capacity of CD4+ T cells underlies the impaired DTH reactivity in old mice. *Mech. Ageing Dev*, 53,127-139.

[83] Gottesman, S.R., Edington, J.M., Thorbecke, G.J. (1988) Proliferative and cytotoxic immune functions in aging mice. IV. Effects of suppressor cell populations from aged and young mice. *J. Immunol*, 140, 1783-1790.

[84] Burns, E.A., Leventhal, E.A. (2000) Aging, immunity, and cancer. *Cancer Control*, 7, 513-522.

[85] Garkavtsev, I., Hull, C., Riabowol, K. (1998) Molecular aspects of the relationship between cancer and aging: tumor suppressor activity during cellular senescence. *Exp. Gerontol*, 33, 81-94.

[86] VanAman, S.E., Whisler, R.L. (1998) Differential expression of p53 tumor suppressor protein and IL-2 in activated T cells from elderly humans. *J. Interferon Cytokine Res*, 18, 315-320.

[87] Cools, N., Ponsaerts, P., Van Tendeloo, V.F., Berneman, Z.N. (2007) Regulatory T cells and human disease. *Clin. Dev. Immunol*, 89195.

[88] Sakaguchi, S. (2005) Naturally arising Foxp3-expressing CD25+CD4+ regulatory T cells in immunological tolerance to self and non-self. *Nature Immunol*, 4, 345-352.

[89] Fontenot, J.D., Rudensky, A.Y. (2005) A well adapted regulatory contrivance: regulatory T cell development and the forkhead family transcription factor Foxp3. *Nature Immunol*, 4, 331-337.

[90] Gregg, R., Smith, C.M., Clark, F.J., Dunnion, D., Khan, N., Chakraverty, R., et al., (2005) The number of human peripheral blood CD4+ CD25high regulatory T cells increases with age. *Clin. Exp. Immunol*, 140, 540-546.

[91] Nishioka, T., Shimizu, J., Iida, R., Yamazaki, S., Sakaguchi, S. (2006) CD4+CD25+Foxp3+ T cells and CD4+CD25-Foxp3+ T cells in aged mice. *J. Immunol*, 176, 6586-6893.

[92] Tsaknaridis, L., Spencer, L., Culbertson, N., Hicks, K., LaTocha, D., Chou, Y.K., et al., (2003) Functional assay for human CD4+CD25+ Treg cells reveals an age-dependent loss of suppressive activity. *J. Neurosci. Res*, 74, 296-308.

[93] Dejaco, C., Duftner, C., Schirmer, M. (2006) Are regulatory T-cells linked with aging? *Exp. Gerontol*, 41, 339-345.

[94] Ligthart, G.J., Schuit, H.R., Hijmans, W. (1985) Subpopulations of mononuclear cells in ageing: expansion of the null cell compartment and decrease in the number of T and B cells in human blood. *Immunology*, 55, 15-21.

[95] Zharhary, D. (1988) Age-related changes in the capability of the bone marrow to generate B cells. *J. Immunol*, 141, 1863-1869.

[96] Klinman, N.R., Kline G.H. (1997) The B-cell biology of aging. *Immunol. Rev*, 160, 103-114.

[97] Van der Put, E., Sherwood, E.M., Blomberg, B.B., Riley, R.L. (2003) Aged mice exhibit distinct B cell precursor phenotypes differing in activation, proliferation and apoptosis. *Exp. Gerontol*, 38, 1137-1147.

[98] Kudlacek S, Willvonseder R, Stohlawetz P, Hahn P, Pietschmann P. (2000) Immunology and aging. *Aging Male*, 3, 137-142.

[99] Montes, C.L., Maletto, B.A., Acosta Rodriguez, E.V., Gruppi, A., Pistoresi-Palencia, M.C. (2006) B cells from aged mice exhibit reduced apoptosis upon B-cell antigen receptor stimulation and differential ability to up-regulate survival signals. *Clin. Exp. Immunol*, 143, 30-40.

[100] Grubeck-Loebenstein, B. (1997) Changes in the aging immune system. *Biologicals*, 25, 205-208.

[101] Delafuente, J.C. (1985) Immunosenescence. Clinical and pharmacologic considerations. *Med. Clin. North Am*, 69, 475-486.

[102] Weksler, M.E., and Szabo, P. (2000) The effect of age on the B-cell repertoire. *J. Clin. Immunol*, 20, 240-249.

[103] LeMaoult, J., Szabo, P., Weksler, M.E. (1997) Effect of age on humoral immunity, selection of the B-cell repertoire and B-cell development. *Immunol. Rev*, 160, 115-126.

[104] Weksler, M.E. (2000) Changes in the B-cell repertoire with age. *Vaccine*, 18, 1624-1628.

[105] Zhao, K.S., Wang, Y.F., Guéret, R., Weksler, M.E. (1995) Dysregulation of the humoral immune response in old mice. *Int. Immunol*, 7, 929-934.

[106] Kishimoto, S., Tomino, S., Mitsuya, H., Nishimura, H. (1982) Age-related decrease in frequencies of B-cell precursors and specific helper T cells involved in the IgG anti-tetanus toxoid antibody production in humans. *Clin. Immunol. Immunopathol*, 25, 1-10.

[107] Remarque, E.J., van Beek, W.C., Ligthart, G.J., Borst, R.J., Nagelkerken, L., Palache, A.M., et al., (1993) Improvement of the immunoglobulin subclass response to influenza vaccine in elderly nursing-home residents by the use of high-dose vaccines. *Vaccine*, 11, 649-654.

[108] Saurwein-Teissl, M., Lung, T.L., Marx, F., Gschösser, C., Asch, E., Blasko, I., et al., (2002) Lack of antibody production following immunization in old age: association with CD8(+)CD28(-) T cell clonal expansions and an imbalance in the production of Th1 and Th2 cytokines. *J. Immunol*, 168, 5893-5899.

[109] Liu, Y.J., Kanzler, H., Soumelis, V., Gilliet, M. (2001) Dendritic cell lineage, plasticity and cross-regulation. *Nat. Immunol*, 2, 585-589.

[110] Schuurhuis, D.H., Fu, N., Ossendorp, F., Melief, C.J.M. (2006) Ins and outs of dendritic cells. *Int. Arch Allergy Immunol*, 140, 53-72.

[111] Donnini, A., Argentati, K., Mancini, R., Smorlesi, A., Bartozzi, B., Bernardini, G., Provinciali, M. (2002) Phenotype, antigen-presenting capacity, and migration of antigen-presenting cells in young and old age. *Exp. Gerontol*, 37, 1097-1112.

[112] Banchereau, J., Steinman, R.M. (1998) Dendritic cells and the control of immunity. *Nature*, 392, 245-252.

[113] Banchereau, J., Briere, F., Caux, Cl. (2000) Immunobiology of dendritic cells. *Ann. Rev. Immunol*, 18, 767-811.

[114] Brode, S., Macary, P.A. (2004) Cross-presentation: dendritic cells and macrophages bite off more than they can chew! *Immunology*, 112, 345-351.

[115] Fujihashi, K., and McGhee, J.R. (2004) Mucosal immunity and tolerance in the elderly. *Mech. Ageing Dev*, 25, 889-898.

[116] Bhushan, M., Cumberbatch, M., Dearman, R.J., Andrew, S.M., Kimber, I., Griffiths, C.E. (2002) Tumour necrosis factor-alpha-induced migration of human Langerhans cells: the influence of ageing. *Br. J. Dermatol*, 146, 32-40.

[117] Zavala, W.D., Cavicchia, J.C. (2006) Deterioration of the Langerhans cell network of the human gingival epithelium with aging. *Arch Oral. Biol*, 51, 1150-1155.

[118] Stichel, C.C., Luebbert, H. (2007) Inflammatory processes in the aging mouse brain: participation of dendritic cells and T-cells. *Neurobiol. Aging*, 28, 1507-1521.

[119] Agrawal, A., Agrawal, S., Jianing, C., Houfen, S., Osann, K., Gupta, S. (2007) Altered innate immune functioning of dendritic cells in elderly humans: a role of phosphoinositide 3-kinase-signaling pathway. *J. Immunol*, 178, 6912-6922.

[120] Sauter, B., Albert, M.L., Francisco, L., Larsson, M., Somersan, S., Bhardwaj, N. (2000) Consequences of cell death: exposure to necrotic tumor cells, but not primary tissue cells or apoptotic cells, induces the maturation of immunostimulatory dendritic cells. *J. Exp. Med*, 191, 423-434.

[121] Agrawal, A., Agrawal, S., Tay, J., Gupta, S. (2008) Biology of dendritic cells in aging. *J. Clin. Immunol*, 28, 14-20.

[122] Rafi, A., Castle, S.C., Uyemura, K., Makinodan, T. (2003) Immune dysfunction in the elderly and its reversal by antihistamines. *Biomed. Pharmacother*, 57, 246-250.

[123] Uyemura, K., Castle, S.C., Makinodan, T. (2002) The frail elderly: role of dendritic cells in the susceptibility of infection. *Mech. Ageing Dev*, 123, 955-962.

[124] Plowden, J., Renshaw-Hoelscher, M., Gangappa, S., Engleman, C., Katz, J.M., Sambhara, S. (2004) Impaired antigen-induced CD8+ T cell clonal expansion in aging is due to defects in antigen presenting cell function. *Cell Immunol*, 229, 86-92.

[125] Haruna, H., Inaba, M., Inaba, K., Taketani, S., Sugiura, K., Fukuba, Y., et al., (1995) Abnormalities of B cells and dendritic cells in SAMP1 mice. *Eur. J. Immunol*, 25, 1319-1325.

[126] Ogawa, T., Kitagawa, M., Hirokawa, K. (2000) Age-related changes of human bone marrow: a histometric estimation of proliferative cells, apoptotic cells, T cells, B cells and macrophages. *Mech. Ageing Dev*, 117, 57-68.

[127] Thiers, B.H., Maize, J.C., Spicer, S.S., Cantor, A.B. (1984) The effect of aging and chronic sun exposure on human Langerhans cell populations. *J. Invest Dermatol*, 82, 223-226.

[128] Plowden, J., Renshaw-Hoelscher, M., Engleman, C., Katz, J., Sambhara, S. (2004), Innate immunity in aging: impact on macrophage function. *Aging Cell*, 3, 161-167.

[129] Renshaw, M., Rockwell, J., Engleman, C., Gewirtz, A., Katz, J., Sambhara, S. (2002) Cutting edge: impaired Toll-like receptor expression and function in aging. *J. Immunol*, 169, 4697-4701.

[130] Fietta, A., Merlini, C., De Bernardi, P.M., Gandola, L., Piccioni, P.D., Grassi, C. (1993) Non specific immunity in aged healthy subjects and in patients with chronic bronchitis. *Aging (Milano)*, 5, 357-361.

[131] Ortega, E., Garcia, J.J., De La Fuente, M. (2000) Ageing modulates some aspects of the non-specific immune response of murine macrophages and lymphocytes. *Exp. Physiol*, 85, 519-525.

[132] Conrad, A., Hansmann, C., Engels, I., Daschner, F.D., and Frank, U. (2007) Extract of Pelargonium sidoides (EPs 7630) improves phagocytosis, oxidative burst, and intracellular killing of human peripheral blood phagocytes in vitro. *Phytomedicine*, 14, 46-51.

[133] Mukae, H., Zamfir, D., English, D., Hogg, J.C., van Eeden, S.F. (2000) Polymorphonuclear leukocytes released from the bone marrow by granulocyte colony-stimulating factor: intravascular behavior. *Hematol. J*, 1, 159-171.

[134] Eyles, J.L., Roberts, A.W., Metcalf, D., Wicks. I.P. (2006) Granulocyte colony-stimulating factor and neutrophils-forgotten mediators of inflammatory disease. *Nat. Clin. Pract. Rheumatol*, 2, 500-510.

[135] Terashima, T., Wiggs, B., English, D., Hogg, J.C., van Eeden, S.F. (1996) Human immunodeficiency virus envelope glycoprotein 120 alters sleep and induces cytokine mRNA expression in rats. *Am. J. Physiol*, 271, L587.

[136] Ulich, T.R., del Castillo, J., Busser, K., Guo, K.Z., Yin, S.M. (1989) Acute in vivo effects of IL-3 alone and in combination with IL-6 on the blood cells of the circulation and bone marrow. *Am. J. Pathol*, 135, 663-670.

[137] Terashima, T., English, D., Hogg, J.C., van Eeden, S.F. (1998) Release of polymorphonuclear leukocytes from the bone marrow by interleukin-8. *Blood*, 92, 1062-1069.

[138] Nagel, J.E., Han, K., Coon, P.J., Adler, W.H., Bender, B.S. (1986) Age differences in phagocytosis by polymorphonuclear leukocytes measured by flow cytometry. *J. Leukoc. Biol*, 39, 399-407.

[139] Schröder, A.K., Rink, L. (2003) Neutrophil immunity of the elderly. *Mech. Ageing Dev*, 124, 419-425.

[140] Wenisch, C., Patruta, S., Daxböck, F., Krause, R., Hörl, W. (2000) Effect of age on human neutrophil function. *J. Leukoc. Biol*, 67, 40-45.

[141] Gocer, P., Gurer, U.S., Erten, N., Palanduz, S., Rayaman, E., Akarsu, B., et al., (2005) Comparison of polymorphonuclear leukocyte functions in elderly patients and healthy young volunteers. *Med. Princ. Pract*, 14, 382-385.

[142] Angelis, P., Scharf, S., Christophidis, N. (1997) Effects of age on neutrophil function and its relevance to bacterial infections in the elderly. *J. Clin. Lab. Immunol*, 49, 33-40.

[143] De Martinis, M., Modesti, M., Ginaldi, L. (2004) Phenotypic and functional changes of circulating monocytes and polymorphonuclear leucocytes from elderly persons. *Immunol. Cell Biol*, 82, 415-420.

[144] Lanier, L.L. (1998) NK cell receptors. *Annu. Rev. Immunol*, 16, 359-393.

[145] Whiteside, T.L. (2001) *Curr. Protoc. Immunol*, Chapter 7:Unit 7.7.

[146] Ribeiro-Dias, F., Marzagão Barbuto, J.A., Tsujita, M., Jancar, S. (2000) Discrimination between NK and LAK cytotoxic activities of murine spleen cells by MTT assay: differential inhibition by PGE(2) and EDTA. *J. Immunol. Methods*, 241(1-2), 121-129.

[147] Kaser A, Hava DL, Dougan SK, Chen Z, Zeissig S, Brenner MB, Blumberg RS., (2008) Microsomal triglyceride transfer protein regulates endogenous and exogenous antigen presentation by group 1 CD1 molecules. *Eur. J. Immunol,* 38, 2351-2359.

[148] Mocchegiani, E., Malavolta, M. (2004) NK and NKT cell functions in immunosenescence. *Aging Cell*, 3, 177-184.

[149] Solana, R., Alonso, M.C., Pena, J. (1999) Natural killer cells in healthy aging. *Exp. Gerontol*, 34, 435-443.

[150] Ravaglia, G., Forti, P., Maioli, F., Bastagli, L., Facchini, A., Mariani, E., et al., (2000) Effect of micronutrient status on natural killer cell immune function in healthy free-living subjects aged >/=90 y. *Am. J. Clin. Nutr*, 71, 590-598.

[151] McNerlan, S.E., Rea, I.M., Alexander, H.D., Morris, T.C. (1998) Changes in natural killer cells, the CD57CD8 subset, and related cytokines in healthy aging. *J. Clin. Immunol*, 18, 31-38.

[152] Chidrawar, S.M., Khan, N., Chan, Y.L., Nayak, L., Moss, P.A. (2006) Ageing is associated with a decline in peripheral blood CD56bright NK cells. *Immun. Ageing*, 3, 10.

[153] Chakraborty, A., Chakraborty, N.G., Chattopadhyay, U. (1994) Age related natural killer activity of peripheral blood lymphocytes from healthy subjects and cancer patients. A comparative in vitro study with interleukin-2. *Tumori*, 80, 233-237.

[154] Rukavina, D., Laskarin, G., Rubesa, G., Strbo, N., Bedenicki, I., Manestar, D., et al., (1998) Age-related decline of perforin expression in human cytotoxic T lymphocytes and natural killer cells. *Blood*, 92, 2410-2420.

In: Immunology in Clinic Practice
Editor: Cagatay Oktenli, pp. 47-76
ISBN 978-1-60876-644-4


*Chapter 4*

# IMMUNOLOGY IN CARDIOLOGY AND PULMONARY MEDICINE CLINICS: RECENT PROGRESS

***Cem Barçın[1], Hürkan Kurşaklıoğlu[1] and Arzu Balkan[2]***
1. Department of Cardiology,
Gülhane Militay Medical Academy, Ankara, Turkey
2. Department of Pulmonary Medicine,
Gülhane Militay Medical Academy, Ankara, Turkey

## ABSTRACT

Inflammation seems to be important in both plaque formation and plaque rupture and many actors of innate and acquired immune system, other than T cells and monocytes, play a role in the atherosclerosis. There is growing evidence that cardiac allograft vasculopathy is primarily an immune-related response to transplantation although the mechanisms of cardiac allograft vasculopathy are not revealed completely. Rheumatic fever is the most common example of molecular mimicry in human pathological autoimmunity. Even though the pathogenesis of rheumatic fever is not completely understood, it is clear that an exacerbated immune response to bacterial antigens in susceptible hosts leads to autoimmune attack to several tissues and, in rheumatic heart disease patients; this triggers an inflammatory response to heart tissue, probably caused by molecular mimicry between group-A streptococcus antigens and heart tissue proteins. Pulmonary immune response induced by antigens divided into 3 phases. These are cognitive phase (defining and processing the antigen), activation phase (proliferation and differentiation of suitable lymphocytes to specific immune cells) and effector phase (regulation of immune responses of specific effectors lymphocytes to eliminate the foreign antigen).

**Keywords:** Atherorosclerosis; plaque formation; cardiac allograft vasculopathy; rheumatic heart disease; lung immunology

# INTRODUCTION

Atherorosclerosis is the leading cause of mortality and morbidity in developed and developing countries. It may be described as a chronic disease of the vessel wall with two main characteristic hallmarks: lipid retention and inflammation [1, 2]. This inflammation is regulated by a complex interplay of innate and acquired immune systems in both early and late stages of atherosclerosis [2]. The initial step in atherosclerosis is probably the accumulation of low density lipoprotein (LDL) cholesterol in the intima of the arteries [4]. It is supposed that endothelial dysfunction or disintegrity precedes this process and allows the LDL particles to travel through the endothelium [3]. Within the arterial wall, LDL particles undergo modification by enzymes and oxygen radicals and transform into proinflammatory particles [4]. These modified LDL particles play a role in the expression of adhesion molecules by the endothelial cells. They also stimulate vascular smooth muscle cells (SMCs) to release chemokines and chemoattractants [5]. All of these steps allow monocytes and T cells, the two major actors of atherosclerosis, to accumulate in the stimulated sites of the arterial wall [6]. These infiltrated monocytes differantiate into foam cells after they uptake the lipids. These are the characteristic steps in the early phase of plaque formation which is also called as fatty streak and can be found in the very early ages of life. These preliminary lesions may progress into complex plaques which narrow the arterial lumen under the influence of many different environmental and genetic risk factors. According to the vessels that are affected, this may result in coronary, renal, limb and/or cerebral ischemia. These plaques may undergo rupture which may lead acute coronary syndromes. Inflammation seems to be important in both plaque formation and plaque rupture and many actors of innate and acquired immune system, other than T cells and monocytes, play a role in the atherosclerosis.

Cells and mediators of the immune system are major contributers of atherosclerotic plaque. These plaques in humans contain blood-borne inflammatory and immune cells, vascular endothelial cells, smooth muscle cells, extracellular matrix, lipids and acellular lipid rich debris [7]. The first steps in human atherogenesis remain at least partly, speculative. However, under the influence of an atherogenic diet, that is typically rich in cholesterol and saturated fat, small lipoprotein particles accumulate in the intima. These lipoprotein particles bind to the the proteoglycans of the extracellular matrix. This binding seems to be responsible from the prolonged residence time for lipoproteins in addition to increased susceptibility of them for oxidative changes [8]. Enzymes including NADH/NADPH oxidase, lipooxygenase, myeloperoxidase contribute to oxidative stres in plaques and convert LDL to oxidized LDL (oxLDL) [9-12]. This process is critical in terms of the pathogenesis of early atherosclerosis as it initiates recruitment and activation of immune cells in atherosclerotic plaques.

# IMMUNITY IN ATHEROSCLEROSIS

## Role of Innate Immunity

Two dominant immune cell types in atherosclerotic plaques are monocytes and T lymphocytes. Early after lipid accumulation, modified lipoproteins become capable of inducing cytokine and chemokine expression [2,13]. The secretion of these mediators induces endothelial cells to express adhesion molecules which regulate the adhesion of monocytes and T-lymphocytes to the endothelium. Animal studies show that these adhesion molecules participate in the formation of fatty streaks, the very first stage of atheroma [14]. Genetically altered mice that are deficient for two adhesion molecules, endothelial-cell selectin (E-selectin) and platelet selectin (P-selectin), have reduced severity of atherosclerosis [14]. Important adhesion molecules which participate in leukocyte-endothelial adhesion include L-selectin, E selectin and P-selectin expressed by leukocytes, endothelial cells and platelets, respectively [14-17]. In addition, vascular cell adhesion molecule 1 (VCAM1) and intercellular adhesion molecule 1 (ICAM-1) are expressed by the endothelial cells and also play an important role in leukocyte-endothelial cell interaction [18,19].

In addition to the adhesion molecules, several chemokines, which are chemoattractant cytokines produced by vascular cells, guide the immune cells to penetrate the endothelial leyer and enter the arterial wall. There are two groups of chemokines as a characteristic of the early atheroma. One such molecule, CC-chemokine ligand 2 (CCL2), is produced by the endothelium in response to oxidized lipoprotein and other stimuli. Experiments on knockout mice show that CCL2 and its receptor CC-chemokine receptor 2 (CCR2) have a crucial role in atherosclerosis [20,21]. CCL2 (or monocyte chemoattractant protein-1 (MCP-1)) selectively targets the chemotaxis of monocytes. Absence of CCL2 and CCR2 limits the the entry of these cells into arterial intima and inhibits plaque formation. Several other chemokines are also released by macrophages or other vascular cells such as T-cell attractants CCL5, CXC chemokine ligand 10, CXCL 11, mast-cell attractant CCL11 [22-24]. Fractalkine ($CX_3$-chemokine ligand 1) is another cell surface-bound-chemokine that involves in the migration of monocytes into the atherosclerotic plaque [24-27]. Different lymphocyte-selective chemokines (IP-10, I-TAC, and MIG) were also found in atherosclerotic plaques [28].

Macrophages are the dominant cell type in plaques. These macrophages are capable of accumulating the oxidized and modified lipoproteins and become foam cells, the lipid-laden macrophage. Scaveneger receptors on the macrophages seem to mediate phagocytosis and lysosomal degradation of lipoprotein particles [29-30]. These receptors are a family of proteins that include CD36, CD68, CCL16, lectin-type oxLDL receptor 1 (LOX1), scavenger receptor (SR) A and B1 [29,30] .

Once macrophages become foam cells, they replicate. Macrophage-colony stimulating factor (M-CSF), interleukin 3 (IL-3) and granulocyte-macrophage colony stimulating factor (GM-CSF) have important role in this replication. Absence of functional M-CSF has retarded fatty lesion development in mice [28]. On the other hand, lack of LDL receptors is not related with foam cell formation.

Another type of actor in atherosclerosis is Toll-like receptors (TLR). These transmembrane proteins play a crucial role in both innate and acquired immune systems and amino acid sequence eleven TLRs have been identified in mammals [31-34]. In human atherosclerotic plaques, elevated mRNA and and protein levels of TLR1, TLR2 and TLR4 have been found [35,36]. TLR2 and TLR4 are expressed mainly by macrophages ad endothelial cells in plaques [37]. In contrast, expression of TLR2 and TLR4 is very low in endothelial cells of normal arterial segments. Events that are mediated by TLRs induce inflammation. TLRs recognize pathogen associated molecular paterns on the surface of pathogens [38]. Especially TLR2 and TLR4 recognize a broad range of surface molecular patterns such as microbial components and heat schock proteins (HSPs). Furthermore there is evidence that endogenous HSP60 and oxLDL can promote inflammation via binding TLR4-CD14 complex [39-41]. Four adaptor molecules have been shown to bind TLRs, resulting in activation and nuclear translocation of nuclear factor kappa beta (NF-κB). NF-κB activates IL-6, IL1β and tumor necrosis factor-α (TNF-α), increases expression of adhesion molecules (ICAM-1, VCAM-1 and selectin), and increases chemokine release such as MCP-1 and IL-8 [42]. Animal studies suggest that genetic deficiency in TLR4 or its signal-transducing adaptor molecule myeloid differentiation primary-response gene 88 (MyD88) reduces the formation of atherosclerotic plaques [43-44].

## Role of Adaptive Immunity

All of the above events represent the innate immunity, which is not dependent to antigen stimulation and largely involve monocyte-derived macropahages. In addition to innate immunity, huge body of evidence suggests the role of adaptive (antigen-specific) immunity in atheroma formation and especially in plaque progression [2,45].

In human atherosclerotic plaques the predominant cell type is monocyte derived macrophages. Almost 10% of cells are $CD3^+$ T cells and most of the remaining is smooth muscle cells. In addition to these cells, small number of mast cells, B lymphocytes and dendritic cells are also found in plaques [7]. Mononuclear phagocytes are the major antigen presenting cells in plaques. Antigens for stimulating this adaptive immune response include modified lipoproteins such as oxLDL, HSPs, $beta_2$ glycoprotein Ib, and other antigens derived from infectious agents such as Chlamydia pneumonia [46,47]. These antigens are presented to the T lymphcytes. Advanced plaques contain both CD4+ and CD8+ T cells [7]. Most T cells in plaques, resembling the composition in peripheral blood, are αβ T cells and antigen recognition involves these αβ TCR (T cell receptor) CD4+ T cells [46].

Antigen presenting cells internalize oxLDL via scavenger-receptor pathway [50]. These cells present some fragments of oxLDL to CD4+ cells. These CD4+ lymphocytes probably recognize especially ApoB derived oligopeptides [46]. Upon activation T cells can secrete different cytokines that can modulate atherogenesis. CD4+ T cells have subtypes with different dominant functions. Most of them are T helper 1 ($T_H1$) subtype which secretes proinflammatory cytokines such as interferon gamma, IL-12, IL15, IL 18, lymphotoxin, CD40 ligand, and TNF-α. These cytokines promote atherogenesis as well as lead to plaque destabilization and increased thrombogenity [51]. A number of studies have shown the predominance of $T_H1$ cells within human and mouse atherosclerotic lesions [52,53]. T helper 2 ($T_H2$) subtype, on the other hand, can inhibit inflammation via different cytokines such as IL 10 or IL 4 [54]. As, the dominat subtype of these two T cells is the former one, it may be concluded that $T_H1$ cells play a major role in atherosclerosis. Different studies suggest that in hypercholesterlemic mice lacking $T_H1$ induced cytokines or their receptors, such as interferon gamma (IFN-γ), IL 12, IL18, TNF atherosclerosis is reduced [55-58]. In addition, inhibition of $T_H1$ cells by pentoxifyllin gave a similar result [59]. BALB/c mice which are prone to $T_H2$ type immune response are resistant to atherogenesis even under high cholesterol diet, supporting the protective role of $T_H2$ cells further [60]. On the other hand there is still controversy with the idea that $T_H1$ cytokines promote paque formation whereas $T_H2$ cytokines reduce it. Although some studies showed the protective role of IL4, a prototype of $T_H2$

cytokines, others showed reduced plaque formation in the absence of IL-4 and interleukin-12 in the progression of atherosclerosis in apolipoprotein E-deficient mice [50,57,61].

In addition to cytokines, cell surface proteins CD40 and CD40 ligand have proatherogenic properties [50]. Almost all of the critical players in atherosclerosis, such as macrophages, T-lymphocytes, endothelial cells, SMCs and platelets express CD40 and CD40 ligand [62,63]. The results of CD40 ligation in these cells are the secretion of cytokines and matrix metalloproteinases (MMPs), and the expression of adhesion molecules [64]. Also, in macrophages, CD40 ligation causes expression of the tissue factor, an important molecule in the coagulation cascade.

## Role of Humoral Immunity

Recent studies have showed the role of humoral immunity in atherosclerosis. Antibodies aganist oxLDL of IgM and IgG type were found in both human and animal plasma and these antibodies were found to make complexes with the antigen, oxLDL, found in atherosclerotic plaques. These anti-oxLDL antibodies were demonstrated to extend atherosclerosis in different studies [65,66]. Anti-oxLDL antibodies also recognize the phosphoryhcholine in the cell wall of Streptococcus pneumonia [67]. Interestingly, immunization of LDL cholesterol receptor deficient mice with a pneumococcal vaccine reduced the extend of atherosclerosis [68].

Antibodies aganist HSPs are also interesting in terms of evidence in the role of humaral immunity in atherosclerosis. HSP 60 and 65 are immunogenic proteins found in atherosclerotic plaques and they play a role in the progression of atheroma [69]. Antibodies aganist these HSP have been found in animals with atherosclerosis and correlated with disease progression [70]. Interestingly, antibodies against mycobacteria HSP 65 have been associated with carotid coronary atherosclerosis and myocardial infarction [71].

The sequential homology between infecting microorganism HSP and human HSP suggest that antibodies aganist a pathogen microorganism could also commence autoimmune response that increase atherosclerosis [72,73].

Infections with microorganisms that contain homologue HSP proteins can initiate an autoimmune response by molecular similarity [72-74]. On the other hand antibiotic therapy for Chlamydia pneumoniae did not reduce cardiovascular mortality or morbidity [75]. Immunization aganist oxLDL and HSP65 in order to prevent atherosclerosis showed different effects as some of them was protective but others were detrimental [76-80].

Other members of humoral immunity that participates in atherosclerotic process are antiphospholipid antibodies [81,82]. These antibodies are produced aganist cardiolipin antigens or proteins linked to cardiolipin such as beta2-glycoprotein. These antibodies were shown to increase the expression of adhesion molecules (ICAM-1 and VCAM-1) by endothelial cells, and increase production of IL6 [83]. It has been demonstrated that immunisation of LDL cholesterol receptor deficient mice with cardiolipin results in high anticardiolipin antibody titres and accelerated atherosclerosis [84]. Clinical studies have demonstrated the association of antibodies against beta2-gp1 with coronary artery disease [85,86].

## Protective Immunity Aganist Atherosclerosis

In contrast to dominant action of local cellular immunity in favor of increased atherosclerosis, IL-10 and transforming growth factor-β (TGF-β) exert a constitutive anti-inflammatory and atheroprotective actions [87]. Deficiency of IL-10 caused increased number of fatty streaks in mice under high cholesterol diet [88].

Galigiuri et al. [89] showed in apolipoprotein E knockout mice that IL-10 deficiency plays a deleterious role in atherosclerosis. This deficiency caused both increased lesion development in early phase. Furthermore it was associated with enhanced proteolytic and procoagulant activity in the late stage of atherosclerosis. These data indicated that IL-10 may reduce atherogenesis and improve the stability of plaques. TGF-β, on the other hand, inhibits proliferation and migration, as well as expression of adhesion molecules involved in leukocyte recruitment in endothelial cell cultures [90]. In addition, TGF-β has a range of direct effects on immune cells in culture, including inhibition of foam cell formation in cultured macrophages [91].

## Immunity in Plaque Stability

As huge body of evidence indicates, plaque stability is of paramount importance in the clinical scenario of acute coronary syndromes, the leading cause of mortality and morbidity in developed and developing countries. Unstable plaques can be defined as plaques that are prone to rupture as a result of which thrombotic occlusion of the artery occur. Structure of fibrous cap of the plaque, cellularity and the number of immun cells in plaques, neovascularization, matrix remodelling, degree of apoptosis are among the important features concerning the stability of the paque [92,93]. Immune sytem is involved in almost all of these steps especially in matrix degradation and apoptosis [94]. The thinner the fibrous cap the easier the process of plaque rupture. The balance between the collagen synthesis and degradation determines the durability of the fibrous cap. In this way, inflammatory cytokines can regulate both the expression of genes that direct interstitial collagen synthesis and MMPs required [94]. Vascular SMCs are the main source of collagen synthesis in arterial wall. Matrix metalloproteinases, on the other hand, are a group of proteinases that degrade fibrillar collagen type I and III, proteoglycans, collagen, and elastin, which are all substantial constituents of the fibrous atherosclerotic cap [95]. In general, inflammatory cytokines such as interferon gamma, decreasese collagen synthesis and increases apaptosis of VSMCs [96]. Sudies suggest that macrophage derived MMPs are increased in unstable plaques [97]. In addition, MMPs can also enhance the activity of some cytokines such as TNF α, IL 1β as well as the adhesion and the aggregation of platelets [95,98-100]. Despite these findings the role of MMPs in atherosclerosis and plaque stability is inconclusive. Apperantly different type of MMPs may have different actions. Overexpression of MMP-1but deficiency of MMP-2 has the similar effect and both conditions are associated with less collagen accumulation in atheroma [101,102]. Paradoxically, decrease in plaque volume does not mean that increase in plaque stability.In fact, degradation of plaque matrix including SMCs is suggested to decrease plaque stability [103]. Further studies are needed to clarify the exact role of both MMPs and VSMCs in atherosclerosis and plaque stability.

In addition to SMC replication, apoptosis of these cells may also participate in complication of the atherosclerotic plaque [104,105]. Apoptosis in plaques is associated with the accumulation of inflammatory cells and inflammatory cytokines (TNF-α and IL-1β). T cell populations can lead to death of the SMC [104,106,107]. Decrease in SMCs in plaques may weaken the plaque and cause vulnerability for plaque rupture [108,109]. Furthermore vasvular SMC apoptosis may also cause release of inflammatory cytokines (IL-1α, IL-8, and MCP-1), which in turn causes macrophage recruitment into the lesions [110]. Macrophages are major players of immune system in plaque vulnerability. It has recently been shown that macrophage derived MMPs, which is a marker of plaque vulnerability, is increased in human unstable carotid plaques [97]. Unstable plaques were also found to have increased amounts of apoptotic celss including macrophages and vascular SMCs [110,111]. IL-10, which is known as protective in atherogenesis acts aganist apoptosis and suggested to increase plaque stability [112].

In addition to macrophages $T_H1$ subtype of T cells have major contribution to plaque instability especially via IFN-γ. This cytokine enhance the recruitment of macrophages and T cells to the atheromatous area, the formation of foam cells and the activation of antigen presenting cells [113]. They also cause a positive feedback by increasing the secretion of $T_H1$ promoting cytokines, all of which contribute to plaque destabilization. Furthermore IFN-γ makes the plaque more vulnerable by decreasing collagen synthesis and incresing apoptosis and matrix degradation. In immune cell family some minorities also play a role in plaque destabilization. Mast cells are effective in both MMP production and apoptosis resulting in weakening fibrous cap. Mast cells and mast cell derived MMP-1 has been found at the shoulder region of the fibrous cap where the rupture occurs [114,115]. These cells secrete IL-6, IFN-γ and TNF-α all of which increase and activate MMPs [116]. Mast cells, with secreting chymase, also accelerate apoptosis by activating a couple of key molecules such as caspase-8 and caspase 9. Another minority, platelets, also participate in atherosclerosis and plaque unstability [117].

Platelets store and secrete different inflammatory mediators such as IL-7, soluable CD40 ligand. They also induce macrophages, granulocytes and endothelial cells to express inflammatory sustances such as TNF-α [118-120]. Platelets also induce NFκB and increase the production of several chemokines [121]. It has also been shown that platelet-derived prostoglandin E activates monocytes [122].

## Immunity in Cardiac Allograft Vasculopathy

Cardiac transplantation is a mainstream treatment for patients with refractory end-stage heart disease. Although the survival rates for cardiac transplant patients improve, the long-term complications of the procedure are becoming apparent. Cardiac allograft vasculopathy (CAV) characterized as chronic allograft rejection is one of these long term complications [123]. It is estimated that 15% to 20% of cardiac transplant recipients will develop CAV each year after transplantation. CAV is time dependent. CAV is detectable by angiography in 8% of survivors within the first year, in 32% within the first 5 years, and in 43% within the first 8 years after heart transplantation [124]. It may be unrecognized because of a lack of sensitive screening techniques early after heart transplantation.

CAV is characterized as a diffuse and accelerated form of obliterative coronary artery disease. It differs from the classic atheromatous disease and affects both the arterial and venous structures of the allograf. It can also extend to the donor aortic root without involvement of blood vessels outside the transplanted organ [125]. Although CAV has a multifactorial etiology, there is growing evidence that CAV is primarily an immune-related response to transplantation [125,126].

The hallmark lesion of CAV is a diffuse, concentric fibrous intimal hyperplasia that appears along the entire length of the affected vessels in both the epicardial and intramyocardial arteries and also veins of the transplanted heart [127]. In addition to endothelial cells, lymphocytes, and SMCs, monocyte-derived macrophages play a critical role in CAV. The cascade of growth factor and cytokine release results in the recruitment of SMCs from the media to the intima. Subsequently, the proliferation of SMCs and the secretion of extracellular matrix proteins are seen. The internal elastic lamina and media are usually intact. Changes in the intima can be seen as early as 6 months after transplantation [128]. The smaller branches are often occluded before the larger epicardial arteries.

## Immunologic Characteristics

Irrespective of the initial specific immune-mediated injury, the cascade of activation and dysfunction of the arterial endothelium appears to be a physiologically nonspecific inflammatory response [129]. Although the exact pathogenesis of CAV remains to be established, several lines of data suggest that it is almost universally accepted as a chronic alloimmunologic response to the transplanted organ. Limitation of the proliferative vascular disease to the allograft arterial and venous tree, diffuse nature of allograft vascular involvement in most of the times, the development of CAV in cardiac allografts of animal models with some histocompatibility mismatch, and the lack of development in isografts support the immunologic hypothesis of CAV development [130]. Acute rejection as a cause or risk factor for CAV has been investigated by several authors [131,132]. But there is a substantial knowledge about episodes of acute rejection is not associated with the development of CAV [131,133].

After cardiac transplantation, humoral or more importantly, cellular mediated alloreactivity to human leukocyte antigen (HLA) and vascular endothelial cell antigens are potential sources of endothelial damage. However, HLA class I or class II mismatching was not found to be associated with posttransplant coronary atherosclerosis in a large, single-center study [134]. Several studies point to a cell-mediated immune response [135-137].

## Cellular Mediated Rejection

The coronary endothelial cells of the allograft are the first donor cells to be recognized by the recipient's immune system [138,139]. They express both MHC class I and class II antigens constitutively in response to cytokines [138,139].

Three distinct mechanisms were shown to elucidate this allorecognition: direct, indirect, and semidirect pathways. In direct pathway, the major stimulus for cellular response to transplanted organs is recognition of foreign MHC molecules on the surface of donor cells by recipient dendritic cells (DCs) (allorecognition) and mediates acute rejection [140]. The recipient's DCs are the major cells that recognize MHC molecules on the allograft endothelium [141]. DCs stimulate T lymphocytes (1 dendritic cell may stimulate up to 1000 T lymphocytes) [141]. The activated lymphocytes (CD4 and CD8) adhere to graft endothelial cells and invade the vessel wall. In addition, it has been previously reported that allogenic lymphocytes are capable of activating coronary endothelium [129].

The indirect pathway occurs when donor antigens are internalized, processed, and presented by host DCs [141]. Host DCs frequently adhere to allograft endothelial cells, invade the tissue, capture foreign antigens, and present alloantigens to native host T cells. It mediates chronic rejection/transplant arteriosclerosis. The impact of the recently described semidirect pathway of immune recognition for CAV is unknown [142].

Although the CD4+ allorecognition pathway is required for CAV development, the CD8+ pathway may act to increase the severity of CAV [143]. In a previous study [144], in contrast to the CD4+ T-cell–depleted recipient, hearts transplanted into CD8+ T-cell-depleted rats developed CAV.

In addition, human graft endothelial cells can directly activate allogeneic host T cells through direct presentation of foreign HLA molecules and costimulators [145]. High HLA-DR expression were reported on the endothelium of human coronary allografts [146] These endothelial cells could stimulate foreign T cells *in vitro* [146]. Severe CAV is positively correlated with a higher degree of HLA mismatch and HLA-DR matching is a strong and independent predictor of outcome [147,148].

Plasma levels of oxLDL correlate with the extent of angiographic CAV [149]. Also, adhesion molecules plays an important role in interaction of inflammatory cells with vascular wall cells. In cardiac transplant patients, expression of vascular adhesion molecules such as VCAM-1, ICAM-1, and ELAM-1 on endothelial cells and medial SMCs has been reported [150]. It has been reported that an early ICAM-1 expression could be correlated to early development of angiographically visible CAV [151].

Immunoreactivity for endothelin-1 in coronary arteries of CAV patients were reported to be higher than normal coronary arteries [152]. Endothelial dysfunction is also associated with increased myocardial endothelin mRNA expression after transplantation [153]. TNF-α has been reported to destabilize mRNA message for eNOS and the exposure of endothelial cells to TNF- α reduces NO synthesis and bioactivity [154,155]. Moreover, TNF-α may induce the endothelial expression of inducible Nitric oxide synthase [153]. Hepatocyte growth factor (HGF) has an anti-apoptotic effect on endothelial cells and augments angiogenesis. Thus, CAV might be prevented and allograft survival might prolong [156,157]. The circulating levels of HGF are inversely correlated with angiographically silent CAV.

The activation of T cells by lymphocytes and macrophages requires an interaction between CD28 on the T cell and B7 on the target cell [158]. Human endothelial cells do not express B7, and therefore, an alternative ligand interaction such as CD2-LFA-3 may provide this co-stimulation [159]. The secondary signals derived from these alternative ligand interactions differ in their long-term responses and might be susceptibility to chronic immunosuppression.

The development of clinically evident CAV depends on the interplay between the lesion-formation responses of the allograft to injury versus the adaptive process of vascular remodeling [160-162]. The expansion of the intimal lesion eventually overcomes the capacity of the vessel and creates a vessel stenosis (compensatory enlargement remodeling). There may be a possible lack of compensatory dilation of the vessel wall over time [163]. However, dilated angiopathy, a specific subtype of CAV, might be an example of overcompensating positive remodeling [164].

## Humoral Mediated Rejection

The humoral arm of the immune system in the pathogenesis of CAV is poorly understood in cardiac transplant recipients [165]. It has been reported that antibodies against non-HLA endothelial cell antigens has been associated with a higher incidence of CAV during the first year after transplantation [166]. In 1 to 2 years after transplantation, elevated levels of IgM antibodies against endothelial cell peptides were reported in patients with rapidly progressive CAV [167,168].

Interestingly, approximately 10% to 20% of patients have episodes of hemodynamic compromise with no evidence of cellular rejection in endomyocardial biopsies but also they have alloantibodies predominantly specific for donor graft HLA class I and class II molecules [169-173]. The association between antibody deposition in the cardiac allograft and an increased incidence of CAV in those patients with antibody deposition was demonstrated by immunohistochemistry [172]. In heart transplant patients, it was reported that the HLA-DR mismatch has a significant effect on long-term survival and cardiac allograft vasculopathy, whereas HLA-A and HLA-B show no such correlation [148,156].

Somewhere between 15% and 82% of patients will develop detectable levels of circulating antibodies by 6 months after transplant [174]. The majority of patients will remain asymptomatic and some will probably develop acute antibody-mediated rejection. Monitoring of these donor-specific HLA antibodies on a routine basis may be useful in preventing and diagnosis of rejection episodes before clinical manifestations of irreversible organ damage [175,176].

Circulating antibodies mediate rejection through complement activation and fixation on graft endothelium [170,177]. In this way, the terminal components of complement C5b-C9 (membrane attack complex (MAC)) can cause significant injury to cardiac allografts. MAC stimulates the translocation of P-selectin from platelet a granules to the plasma membrane and the secretion of mediators from storage granules [178,179]. Similarly, in the endothelial cells, MAC causes the translocation of P selectin from Weibel-Palade bodies to plasma membrane and the release of von Willebrand factor [180]. In addition, MAC-stimulated endothelial cells have been found to synthesize and release IL-1 and tissue factor [181]. These responses to MAC cause the transformation of an anticoagulant situation to a procoagulant situation.

The endothelial cells, fibroblasts, and myocytes are among the cells that are capable of synthesizing several complement components, especially C6 [182]. C6 produced by the macrophages caused extensive endothelial injury and platelet aggregation and it can be a significant factor in tissue injury as exemplified by allograft rejection. Limited concentrations of C6 can thwart lysis of nucleated target cells in vitro. Because multiple MAC lesions are required to cause lysis of nucleated cells and MAC channels have a half-life of approximately 1 minute on nucleated cells [183]. Complement 1-q can increase platelet procoagulant activity, release several vasoactive substances and growth factors [184].

Although the development of posttransplant allograft rejection episodes strongly correlates with the development of anti-HLA alloantibodies, antiendothelial antibodies produced by cardiac allograft recipients, using sodium dodecyl sulfate–polyacrylamide gel electrophoresis were also investigated and it was showed that the presence of peptide-specific antiendothelium antibodies were strongly associated with the development of CAV [167].

There is accumulating evidence that the innate immune response via TLR signaling is involved in the immune recognition of allografts [185,186]. It has been reported that increased TLR-4 gene expression in circulating monocytes was associated with allograft coronary endothelial dysfunction [187]. In an experimental model of orthotopic aortic allograft transplantation, ischemia and reperfusion result in endothelial injury and transplant vasculopathy [188]. Endothelial progenitors in human transplanted heart are significantly decreased in the circulation, whereas recipient endothelial cells are increased in coronary arteries of patients with CAV [189,190].

In patients with CAV, immunosuppressive agents (rapamycin and FK506) could led to a significant improvement in short-term survival, although they did not change the long-term death rate significantly [191]. The use of mycophenolate mofetil and proliferation signal inhibitors (everolimus and sirolimus) reduce intimal thickening and might reduce antibody production [192,193]. The prophylaxis and modification of numerous risk factors also might be helpful in the posttransplant management of heart transplant recipients to prevent the initiation and progression of CAV.

## IMMUNITY IN RHEUMATIC HEART DISEASE

Even though the pathogenesis of RF is not completely understood, it is clear that an exacerbated immune response to bacterial antigens in susceptible hosts leads to autoimmune attack to several tissues and, in rheumatic heart disease (RHD) patients; this triggers an inflammatory response to heart tissue, probably caused by molecular mimicry between group-A streptococcus antigens and heart tissue proteins [194]. Abnormal humoral and cellular immune response play an important role in the development of RHD [195-197].

Group A streptococci contain M, T, and R surface proteins and lipoteichoic acid, which are involved in bacterial adherence to pharyngeal epithelial cells [195,196]. The M protein is the most important antigenic structure of the bacterium. This protein shares structural homology with human proteins such as cardiac myosin, tropomyosin, keratin, laminin, vimentin, and several valvular proteins [195-199]. The most important heart autoantigen is cardiac myosin in all of these cardiac proteins [200].

HLA-DR7 is the allele most consistently associated with RHD. The association of HLA-DR7 with different DQ-B or DQ-A alleles seems to be associated with the development of multiple valvular lesions in RHD patients [194-196]. Polymorphisms in genes coding for cytokines and other molecules directly involved in the control of immune response have been also described. Polymorphisms of TGF-β1, immunoglobulin and TNF-α gene were associated with susceptibility to RF development.

## Humoral Immune Response

Autoimmune response is triggered by molecular mimicry between antigens of group-A streptococcus and specific human tissues. Antibodies associated with carditis were first described in 1945 by Calveti. Kaplan and Svec discovered immunoglobulins and complement bound to the myocardium of acute RF patients [194,195]. Subsequent to this discovery, several investigators have focused on identifying the crossreactive antigens that induced humoral immun response. Streptococcal M proteins are the most responsible for crossreactivity. Human cardiac proteins (myosin and vimentin) seem to be the major crossreactive antigens. Especially S. Pyogenes M5 (type 5) protein appears to have triggered autoimmun reactins. Another streptococcal antigen capable of eliciting crossreactive antibodies is the N-acetylglucosamine carbohydrate. It was also demonstrated that N-acetylglucosamine antibodies from RF patients crossreacted with cardiac myosin and laminin. These antibodies showed cytotoxic activity against human endothelial cell-lines and reacted with human valvular endothelium and underlying basement membrane [194,195,201].

Consequently, crossreactive antibodies in RHD cause injury to the endothelium and underlying matrix of the valve. In addition, these antibodies lead initial inflammatory response that triggers cellular infiltration. Increased expression of VCAM-1 after binding of crossreactive antibodies to cardiac tissues facilitates cellular infiltration.

## Cellular Immune Response

Cellular immune response began to be investigated approximately 25 years after the description of the crossreactive antibodies in the development of RF. Rheumatic carditis is initially mediated by a humoral immune response and this response facilitates cellular immune response. Consequantly RHD is a T cell mediated autoimmun disease [194,201].

The characteristic sign of acute RHD, the Aschoff body, is formed in the myocardium and/or endocardium. It contains cellular infiltration. In this infiltrate, the main cell is CD4 T lymphocytes but B cells, macrophages, large mononuclear cells, multinucleated cells and PMNLs exist. Stimulated T cell could induce cytotoxic lymphocytic responses [195].

Heart-infiltrating T cell clones simultaneously recognized streptococcal M5 synthetic peptides and heart tissue-derived proteins, indicating crossreactive epitopes [194-196,202]. It has been showed that T cell response to M5 peptides could discriminate between the M protein recognition patterns of severe and mild RHD patients and healthy subjects [202]. Peptides M5 (81-96) and M5 (91-103) were recognized by 46.0% of severe RHD patients and 8.6% of healthy subjects (P=0.0005), and 24.3% of severe RHD and 3.0% of healthy subjects (P=0.01), respectively [194].

## Cytokines in RHD

Some studies showed that TNF-α, IL-1 and IL-2 were overproduced by peripheral mononuclear cells in patients with RHD. Low levels of these cytokines were produced by tonsillar mononuclear cells from the same patients. During the acute phase of RHD, the production of IL-1, TNF-α and IL-2 correlated with the progression of Aschoff nodules in heart lesions. It has been reported that the increased production of IL-2 in chronic RHD patients correlates with the numbers of CD4 and CD25 cells on the periphery [195,196,203].

It has recently been shown that mononuclear cells from heart lesions predominantly secrete IFN-γ and TNF-α in chronic RHD patients. IL-4 positive cells were predominant in the myocardium, whereas IL4-positive cells were scarce in the valves. Consequently myocardium infiltrating T-cell lines produced IL-4 and IL-10, whereas valve-derived T-cell lines did not produce IL-4 and produced less IL-10 than myocardial derived T-cell lines. By contrast, streptococcal M5-antigen-stimulated T-cell lines produced IFN-γ in 85% of cases. The lack of IL-4, a regulatory cytokine, in the valvular tissue is involved in the progression and permanence of these lesions. In addition, the lack of IL-4 probably perpetuates the production of inflammatory cytokines such as TNF-α and IFN-γ [195,196,204].

## Recent Progress in Pulmonary Medicine

We have to examine the psychopathology of the organs in our body to understand their function completely. Basis of their psychopathology is, however, their immunology. Lung immunology behaves differently in healthy individuals and in the diseased lung.

Although environment stimulates the immune system, the main controllers of immunity are the genes. Genes specifically code the cellular surface for antibodies and cytokines. Since genes control immunity, the resulting changes are capable of affecting the immunologic functions. Cancer, allergic diseases and autoimmune can develop as a result of immunological impairments.

Main cells constituting the immune system are T-cells, B-cells, phagocytes, and NK (Natural Killer) cells. Natural host mechanisms involved in the lung immunology can be listed under 9 headlines. These are desquamation of epithelial cells, secretion of the surface of the epithelium, changes in mucus pH, mucosal hum oral immunity, competition with microorganisms of normal flora, mucociliary transport, coughing, reflex, production of surfactant, alveolar macrophages, and migration of neutrophils.

Actively continuing mucociliary function causes microorganisms within the respiratory system to be unable to hold on. Low Ph in mucus prevents bacterial colonization. Basis of the immunity of the respiratory system however, consists of respiratory immunoglobulins. IgA is the secretory immunoglobulin, and the immunoglobulin that iş most abundant in secretions. It directly activated by the complement and ensures the start of the immune response. IgA is the basic immunoglobulin in the upper respiratory tract, and IgG is the basic immunoglobulin in the lower respiratory tract. IgG is found in alveolar fluid. IgG1, G2, and G4 are the order of amounts of IgG types from high to low. They have an important place in the activation of the complement. In addition, there are substances with antibacterial activity [205]. Complement, lysozyme, fibronectin, free fatty acids, surfactant and iron binding proteins like defensins.

There are epithelial cells that perform and important function by acting as a barrier against the spread of microorganisms. While fagocitic cells participate in chemo taxis and production of chemokins, arachidonic acid derivatives like IL-8, macrophage inflammatory protein and GMCSF can regulate the expression of endothelial adhesion molecules that direct PMNL to the lungs.

In bronchoalveolar lavage (BAL), there are remnants of macrophages 85%, lymphocytes 10%, PMNLs 2%, eosinophils, basophiles and epithelial cells, respectively. There are more than 15 million cells in BAL normally. In some lung diseases however, the situation regarding cells is as follows: in lung tuberculosis, involving CD4 T-cells in lymphocytic alveolitis, alveolar interstitial pneumonitis in sarcoidosis, and increase of neutrophils in ARDS are noted [206,207].

Alveolar macrophages are located in the entry of airways. Respiratory system is the first immunity element that bacterial agents encounter. Clinical studies have shown that macrophages are central for the restriction of consequences of bacterial impacts. In elimination, consequences developing against infection mostly depend on the communication between the bacteria entering the lower respiratory system and the pulmonary defense systems.

Antigen must be relieved from the defense of the natural immune system and defeat the surface barriers to reach regional lymph nodes to stimulate a specific response. Antigen can be followed within airways in mucosal lymphatic tissue and alveolar spaces. Antigen is picked from the interstitium and processed in bronchial or lung-related lymph nodes. Antigens can also defeat the epithelial barriers in various ways and enter the regional lymph nodes after being picked up macrophages, and then drained into regional lymph nodes again. Regulation of inflammatory reactions occurs with passage from one side of this broken epithelium to the other side. Interstitial dendritik cells for transport and process take in antigen particles in regional lymph nodes. Antigen can reach the regional lymph nodes directly, and here they are phagocyted by macrophages localized here and submitted to T-and B-lymphocytes; or else, antigen transport occurs after being phagocyted by macrophages in the interstitium. After this processing and introduction procedure is completed and specific T-lymphocyte population and vascular circulations to find antigens. When entry of antigens is continuous, these specific cells come back with the purpose of helping immune reactions. Increase of surface adhesion molecules of endothelial cells and lymphocytes in lungs play a role in the change of location of antigen-specific lymphocytes, that is, their coming back to lungs. Continuous antigen entry ensures coming of memory lymphocytes included in long-term immunity [208].

Antigen processing for specific humoral or cell-mediated responses and long-term immunity can be responsible for the pathogenesis of several known pulmonary diseases like interstitial pneumonitis or hypersensitivity pneumonitis.

Pulmonary immune response induced by antigens divided into 3 phases. These are, Cognitive phase: defining and processing the antigen; Activation Phase, proliferation and differentiation of suitable lymphocytes to specific immune cells; and Effector Phase, regulation of immune responses of specific effectors lymphocytes to eliminate the foreign antigen.

Cognitive Phase: This is the phase for transport and processing the antigen Foreign antigens are frequently found in upper and lower respiratory tracts, including alveoli. Antigens with large particles are cleared away before inducing an immune response. This process requires the system based on monocyte macrophages. Activation phase is known as reproduction and differentiation phase.

Antigen –MHC class II complex binds to CD4+ T-helper lymphocytes and activate these cells. This complex binds particularly to TCR located on the cell surface combined with CD3, which is another floating molecule consisting of alpha and beta chains. CD3-TCR complex render the lymphocyte with antigen specificity thanks to the polymorphism of the variable regions on alpha and beta chains of TCR.

Effector Phase: Extra cellular pathogens (parasites etc) can be controlled with Th-2 mediated humoral response. IL-4 stimulates antibody production and enhances the functions of eosinophils, macrophages and mast cells. Lymphocyte subsets are converted into memory cells following the activation on the other way. This provides for the occurring of a specific immune response with a suitable term [208].

Natural Killers are introduced in the lung lymphocyte population, and their definite roles are not clear. They can be early origins of pro-inflammatory cytokines like INF-alpha or they can play a role in cytotoxic antitumor immunity [209]. In addition, there is another group consisting of gamma-theta chains instead of lymphocytes consisting of alpha and beta chains. Functions of these cells are thought to be no different from those of alpha/beta T-lymphocytes. Circulation of these cells changes in mycobacterium infections, and also plays a role in infections and granulomatous response is involved in the pathogenesis.

Humoral immunity is induced with antigens binding to the receptors of B-lymphocytes originating from bone marrow. IgD and IgM on the surfaces of these lymphocytes behave like receptors. Cell becomes activated with the binding of the antigen and differentiated and proliferated to specific B-lymphocytes. Surface IgD disappears during this process, and capacity of IgG, IgA, IgG and IgM is acquired. Clonal proliferation occurs for the production of specific antibodies.

Patients suffer very frequent upper respiratory tract infections in selective IgA deficiency. Specific proteolytic enzymes against IgA have been found in organisms colonized in upper respiratory tracts. Some gram-negative bacteria (N.Menengiditis, P.Aureginosa, E.Coli, Serratia, and Proteus) can degrade IgA. Bacterial colonization and ability of causing infections increase with the decreasing IgA, and resulting URTI can spread to lower respiratory tract also. Serum proteins enter air spaces in acute lung damage and inactivate surfactant. Alveolar epithelial cells get damaged and new surfactant synthesis is thus impaired. Abnormal surfactant proteins are insufficient in the regulation of lectin or phagocytosis [210].

Severe combined insufficiency results from different genetic defects, and is seen particularly in MCH II disorder of X-linked disorders. Findings are seen after birth and pneumonia and other infections become more frequent. Causative organisms are opportunistic like P.Carinii, Candida and viruses.

In the Wiscott-Aldrich syndrome, which is an X-liked recessive disorder, there is impairment in the humoral component of the acquired immunity. What held responsible from the increase in tendency to infections is the abnormal immunoglobulin metabolism and weak antibody production [211].

AIDS is the most frequent form of cellular immune deficiency. HIV infection causes decrease in T-helper cells and consequently, functional decrease in other cells. B-cell activation and macrophage functions are affected. Microorganism causing pneumonia related to AIDS is S.Pneumonia, and infection is developed in the early stages of the disease related to humoral defects. Decent and specific infections related to defects dependent on cellular mediation develop later [212].

Polymorphnuclear and mononuclear phagocytes and CD4 T-lymphocytes increase in chronic obstructive pulmonary disease; however, the total amount in the body does not change. To the contrary, an amount of B-cells and CD8 T-lymphocytes increases both in lungs and in the entire system. Role of TH 17 newly defined in the immunopathogenesis of COPD is also great [213, 214].

IL 13 is the main actor of the immune system in bronchial asthma. It is responsible for the synthesis of IgE, hyper reactivity of airways and fibrosis. IL 4 also has activity similar to that of IL3, and has the main role in the immunopathogenesis of asthma [215-217].

Sarcoidosis is a typical immunological disease. Start of the inflammatory process in sarcoidosis is characterized with the accumulation of alveolar macrophages activated with the antigen and T-lymphocytes activated with IL-1 secreted by macrophages in the involved organ. The complex relations of mononuclear phagocytic cells, fibroblasts, dentritic cells and other helper cells on the other hand, regulate granulomatous inflammation. Cytokines secreted by these cells are also greatly responsible for the inflammation. Fibrosis in sarcoidosis however, occurs with the resolution of the granuloma or directly with cytokines relased to the medium [218].

## Conclusion

The immune system has been implicated in atherosclerotic plaque formation, through the activation of humoral and cellular immunity [219-221]. The underlying mechanisms are greatly interconnected and as such very complex. Nevertheless, for clinicians it is important have some degree of insight in these immunologic mechanisms in order to interpret the current research advances [222]. Understanding the underlying mechanisms responsible for inflammatory reactions during atherogenesis may help us to develop novel therapeutic strategies to control, treat and prevent atherosclerosis in the future. Cardiac allograft vasculopathy is the leading cause of late morbidity and mortality in heart transplant patients. Recent insights have underscored the fact that innate and adaptive immune responses are involved in the pathogenesis of cardiac allograft vasculopathy [223]. Furthermore, different immune defenses displayed by lungs in different lung diseases indicate that there are many more characteristics of the immune system yet unknown.

## References


[1] Hansson, G.K. (2005) Inflammation, atherosclerosis, and coronary artery disease. *N. Engl. J. Med*, 352, 1685–1695.

[2] Hansson, G.K., Libby, P., Schonbeck, U., Yan, Z.Q. (2002) Innate and adaptive immunity in the pathogenesis of atherosclerosis. *Circ. Res*, 91, 281–291.

[3] Ross, R. (1999) Atherosclerosis--an inflammatory disease. *New Eng. J. Med*, 340, 115-126.

[4] Witztum, J.L., Steinberg, D. (2001) The oxidative modification hypothesis of atherosclerosis: does it hold for humans? *Trends Cardiovasc. Med*, 11, 93–102.

[5] Simionescu, M. (2007) Implications of early structural-functional changes in the endothelium for vascular disease. *Arterioscler. Thromb Vasc. Biol*, 27, 266–274.

[6] Jonasson, L., Holm, J., Skalli, O., Gabbiani, G., Hansson, G.K. (1985) Expression of class II transplantation antigen on vascular smooth muscle cells in human atherosclerosis. *J. Clin. Invest*, 76, 125–131.

[7] Karaduman, M., Oktenli, C., Musabak, U., Sengul, A., Yesilova, Z., Cingoz, F., Olgun, A., Sanisoglu, S.Y., Baysan, O., Yildiz, O., Taslipinar, A., Tatar, H., Kutlu, M., Ozata, M. (2006) Leptin, soluble interleukin-6 receptor, C-reactive protein and soluble vascular cell adhesion molecule-1 levels in human coronary atherosclerotic plaque. *Clin. Exp. Immunol,* 143, 452-457.

[8] Kruth, H.S. (2002) Sequestration of aggregated low-density lipoproteins by macrophages. *Curr. Opin. Lipid*, 13, 483-88.

[9] Heinecke, J.W. (2003) Oxidative stress: new approaches to diagnosis and prognosis in atherosclerosis. *Am. J. Cardiol*, 91, 12A.

[10] Griendling, K.K. (2004) Novel NAD(P)H oxidases in the cardiovascular system. *Heart*, 90, 491-96.

[11] Papaharalambus, C.A., Griendling, K.K. (2005) Basic mechanisms of oxidative stress and reactive oxygen species in cardiovascular injury. *Trends Cardiovasc. Med,* 17, 48-54.

[12] Cubbon, R.M., Kahn, M.B., Wheatcroft, S.B. (2009) Effects of insulin resistance on endothelial progenitor cells and vascular repair. *Clin. Sci. (Lond)*, 117, 173-190.

[13] Hansson, G.K. (2001) Immune mechanisms in atherosclerosis. *Arterioscler. Thromb Vasc. Biol*, 21, 1876-1890.

[14] Dong, Z. M., Chapman, S.M., Brown, A.A., Frenette, P.S., Hynes, R.O., Wagner, D.D. (1998) The combined role of P- and E-selectins in atherosclerosis. *J. Clin. Invest*, 102, 145–152.

[15] McEver, R.P. (1994) Selectins. *Curr. Opin. Immunol*, 6, 75-84.

[16] Moore, K.L., Patel, K.D., Bruehl, R.E., Li, F., Johnson, D.A., Lichenstein, H.S., et al. (1995) P-selectin glycoprotein ligand-1 mediates rolling of human neutrophils on P-selectin. *J. Cell Biol*, 128, 661-671.

[17] Asa, D., Raycroft, L., Ma, L., Aeed, P.A., Kaytes, P.S., Elhammer, A.P., et al. (1995) The P-selectin glycoprotein ligand functions as a common human leukocyte ligand for P- and E-selectins. *J. Biol. Chem*, 270, 11662-11670.

[18] Chuluyan, H.E., Issekutz, A.C. (1993) VLA-4 integrin can mediate CD11/CD18-independent transendothelial migration of human monocytes. *J. Clin. Invest*, 92, 2768-2777.

[19] Springer, T.A. (1994) Traffic signals for lymphocyte recirculation and leukocyte emigration: the multistep paradigm. *Cell*, 76, 301-314.

[20] Boring, L., Gosling, J., Cleary, M., Charo, I. F. (1998) Decreased lesion formation in CCR2-/- mice reveals a role for chemokines in the initiation of atherosclerosis. *Nature*, 394, 894–897.

[21] Gu, L., Okada, Y., Clinton, S.K., Gerard, C., Sukhova, G.K., Libby, P., Rollins, B.J. (1998) Absence of monocyte chemoattractant protein-1 reduces atherosclerosis in low density lipoprotein receptor-deficient mice. *Mol. Cell*, 2, 275–281.

[22] Mach, F., Sauty, A., Iarossi, A.S., Sukhova, G.K., Neote, K., Libby, P., et al. (1999) Differential expression of three T lymphocyte-activating CXC chemokines by human atheroma-associated cells. *J. Clin. Invest*, 104, 1041–1050.

[23] Haley, K.J., Lilly, C.M., Yang, J.H., Feng, Y., Kennedy, S.P., Turi, T.G., et al. (2000) Overexpression of eotaxin and the CCR3 receptor in human atherosclerosis: using genomic technology to identify a potential novel pathway of vascular inflammation. *Circulation*, 102, 2185–2189.
[24] Tacke, F., Alvarez, D., Kaplan, T.J., Jakubzick, C., Spanbroek, R., Llodra, J., et al. (2007) Monocyte subsets differentially employ CCR2, CCR5, and CX3CR1 to accumulate within atherosclerotic plaques. *J. Clin. Invest*, 117, 185-94.
[25] Combadiere, C., Potteaux, S., Gao, J.L., Esposito, B., Casanova, S., Lee, E.J., et al. (2003) Decreased atherosclerotic lesion formation in CX3CR1/apolipoprotein E double knockout mice. *Circulation*, 107, 1009–1016.
[26] Lesnik, P., Haskell, C.A., Charo, I.F. (2003) Decreased atherosclerosis in CX3CR1-/- mice reveals a role for fractalkine in atherogenesis. *J. Clin. Invest*, 111, 333–340.
[27] Charo, I.F., Ransohoff, R.M. (2006) The many roles of chemokines and chemokine receptors in inflammation. *N. Engl. J. Med*, 354, 610-621.
[28] Libby, P. (2002) Inflammation in atherosclerosis. *Nature*, 420, 868-874.
[29] Miller, Y.I., Chang, M.K., Binder, C.J. (2003) Oxidized low density lipoprotein and innate immune receptors. *Curr. Opin. Lipidol*, 14, 437-445.
[30] van Berkel, T.J., Out, R., Hoekstra, M. (2005) Scavenger receptors: friend or foe in atherosclerosis? *Curr. Opin. Lipidol*, 16, 525-534.
[31] Medzhitov, R., Preston-Hurlburt, P., Janeway, C.A., Jr. (1997) A human homologue of the Drosophila Toll protein signals activation of adaptive immunity. *Nature*, 388, 394-397.
[32] Rock, F.L., Hardiman, G., Timans, J.C., Kastelein, R.A., Bazan, J.F. (1998) A family of human receptors structurally related to Drosophila Toll. *Proc. Natl. Acad. Sci. USA*, 95, 588-593.
[33] Abreu, M.T., Fukata, M., Arditi, M. (2005) TLR signaling in the gut in health and disease. *J. Immunol*, 174, 4453-60.
[34] Abreu, M.T., Arditi, M. (2004) Innate immunity and toll-like receptors: clinical implications of basic science research. *J. Pediatr*, 144, 421-429.
[35] Edfeldt, K., Swedenborg, J., Hansson, G.K., Yan, Z.Q. (2002) Expression of toll-like receptors in human atherosclerotic lesions: a possible pathway for plaque activation. *Circulation*, 105, 1158.
[36] Xu, X.H., Shah, P.K., Faure, E., Equils, O., Thomas, L., Fishbein, M.C., et al. (2001) Toll-like receptor-4 is expressed by macrophages in murine and human lipid-rich atherosclerotic plaques and upregulated by oxidized LDL. *Circulation*, 104, 3103-3108.
[37] Yan, Z.Q. (2002) Expression of toll-like receptors in human atherosclerotic lesions: a possible pathway for plaque activation. *Circulation*, 105, 1158–1161.
[38] Oude Nijhuis, M.M., van Keulen, J.K., Pasterkamp, G., Quax, P.H., de Kleijn, D.P. (2007) Activation of the innate immune system in atherosclerotic disease. *Curr. Pharm. Des*, 13, 983-994.
[39] Kurt-Jones, E.A. (2000) Cutting edge: heat shock protein (HSP) 60 activates the innate immune response: CD14 is an essential receptor for HSP60 activation of mononuclear cells. *J. Immunol*, 164, 13–17.
[40] Curtiss, L.K., Tobias, P.S. (2009) Emerging role of Toll-like receptors in atherosclerosis. *J. Lipid Res*, 50, S340-345.

[41] Miller, Y.I., Viriyakosol, S., Binder, C.J., Feramisco, J.R., Kirkland, T.N., Witztum, J.L. (2003) Minimally modified LDL binds to CD14, induces macrophage spreading via TLR4/MD-2, and inhibits phagocytosis of apoptotic cells. *J. Biol. Chem*, 278, 1561–1568.

[42] Edfeldt, K., Swedenborg, J., Hansson, G. K., Yan, Z. Q. (2002) Expression of toll-like receptors in human atherosclerotic lesions: a possible pathway for plaque activation. *Circulation*, 105, 1158–1161.

[43] Michelsen, K.S., Wong, M.H., Shah, P.K., Zhang, W., Yano, J., Doherty, T.M., Akira, S., Rajavashisth, T.B., Arditi, M. (2004) Lack of Toll-like receptor 4 or myeloid differentiation factor 88 reduces atherosclerosis and alters plaque phenotype in mice deficient in apolipoprotein E. *Proc. Natl. Acad. Sci. USA*, 101, 10679-10684.

[44] Bjökbarcka, H., Kunjathoor, V.V., Moore, K.J., Koehn, S., Ordija, J.M., Lee, M.A., et al. (2004) Reduced atherosclerosis in MyD88-null mice links elevated serum cholesterol levels to activation of innate immunity signaling pathways. *Nature Med*, 10, 416–421.

[45] Binder, C.J., Chang, M.K., Shaw, P.X., Miller YI, Hartvigsen K, Dewan A, Witztum JL. (2002) Innate and acquired immunity in atherogenesis. *Nat. Med*, 8, 1218-1224.

[46] Stemme, S., Faber, B., Holm, J., Wiklund, O., Witztum, J.L., Hansson, G.K. (1995) T lymphocytes from human atherosclerotic plaques recognize oxidized low density lipoprotein. *Proc. Natl. Acad. Sci. USA*, 92, 3893–3897.

[47] de Boer, O.J., van der Wal, A.C., Houtcamp, M.A., Ossewaarde, J.M., Teeling, P., Becker, A.E. (2000) Unstable atherosclerotic plaques contain T-cells that respond to Chlamydia pneumoniae. *Cardiovasc. Res*, 48, 402–408.

[48] Palinski, W., Rosenfeld, M.E., Ylaa-Herttuala, S., Gurtner, G.C., Socher, S.S., Butler, S.W., et al. (1989) Low density lipoprotein undergoes oxidative modification in vivo. *Proc. Natl. Acad. Sci. USA*, 86, 1372–1376.

[49] Palinski, W., Horkko, S., Miller, E., Steinbrecher, U.P., Powell, H.C., Curtis, L.K., et al. (1996) Cloning of monoclonal autoantibodies to epitopes of oxidized lipoproteins from apolipoprotein E-deficient mice. Demonstration of epitopes of oxidized low density lipoprotein in human plasma. *J. Clin. Invest*, 98, 800–814.

[50] Hansson, G.K., Libby, P. (2006) The immune response in atherosclerosis: a double-edged sword. *Nat. Rev. Immunol*, 6, 508-519.

[51] Cuneo, A.A., Autieri, M.V. (2009) Expression and function of anti-inflammatory interleukins: the other side of the vascular response to injury. *Curr. Vasc. Pharmacol*, 7, 267-276.

[52] Daugherty, A., Rateri, D.L. (2002) T lymphocytes in atherosclerosis: the yin-yang of Th1 and Th2 influence on lesion formation. *Circ. Res*, 90, 1039-1040.

[53] Liuzzo, G., Kopecky, S.L., Frye, R.L. (1999) Perturbation of the T-cell repertoire in patients with unstable angina. *Circulation*, 100, 2135-2139.

[54] Pinderski, L.J., Fischbein, M.P., Subbanagounder, G., et al. (2002) Overexpression of interleukin-10 by activated T lymphocytes inhibits atherosclerosis in LDL receptor-deficient Mice by altering lymphocyte and macrophage phenotypes. *Circ. Res*, 90, 1064-1071.

[55] Gupta, S., Pablo, A.M., Jiang, X., Wang, N., Tall, A.R., Schindler, C. (1997) IFN-gamma potentiates atherosclerosis in ApoE knock-out mice. *J. Clin. Invest*, 99, 2752–2761.

[56] Buono, C., Come, C.E., Stavrakis, G., Meguire, G.F., Connely, P.W., Lichtman, A.H. (2003) Influence of interferon-gamma on the extent and phenotype of diet-induced atherosclerosis in the LDLR-deficient mouse. *Arterioscler. Thromb. Vasc. Biol*, 23, 454–460.

[57] Davenport, P., Tipping, P. G. (2003) The role of interleukin-4 and interleukin-12 in the progression of atherosclerosis in apolipoprotein E-deficient mice. *Am. J. Pathol*, 163, 1117–1125.

[58] Branen, L., Hovgaard, L., Nitulescu, M., Bengtsson, E., Nilsson, J., Jovinge, S. (2004) Inhibition of tumor necrosis factor-alpha reduces atherosclerosis in apolipoprotein E knockout mice. *Arterioscler. Thromb Vasc. Biol*, 24, 2137–2142.

[59] Laurat, E., Poirier, B., Tupin, E., Caligiuri, G., Hansson, G.K., Bariéty, J., Nicoletti, A. (2001) In vivo downregulation of T helper cell 1 immune responses reduces atherogenesis in apolipoprotein E-knockout mice. *Circulation*, 104, 197–202.

[60] Huber, S.A., Sakkinen, P., David, C., Newell, M. K., Tracy, R.P. (2001) T helper-cell phenotype regulates atherosclerosis in mice under conditions of mild hypercholesterolemia. *Circulation*, 103, 2610–2616.

[61] King, V.L., Szilvassy, S J., Daugherty, A. (2002) Interleukin-4 deficiency decreases atherosclerotic lesion formation in a site-specific manner in female LDL receptor-/- mice. *Arterioscler. Thromb Vasc. Biol*, 22, 456–461.

[62] Mach, F. (1997) Functional CD40 ligand is expressed on human vascular endothelial cells, smooth muscle cells, and macrophages: implications for CD40-CD40 ligand signaling in atherosclerosis. *Proc. Natl. Acad. Sci. USA*, 94, 1931–1936.

[63] Henn, V., Slupsky, J., Grafe, M., Anagnastopoulos, I., Forster, R., et al. (1998) CD40 ligand on activated platelets triggers an inflammatory reaction of endothelial cells. *Nature*, 391, 591–594.

[64] Mach, F., Schoenbeck, U., Bonnefoy, J.-Y., Pober, J., Libby, P. (1997) Activation of monocyte/macrophage functions related to acute atheroma complication by ligation of CD40: induction of collagenase, stromelysin, and tissue factor. *Circulation*, 96, 396–399.

[65] Salonen, J.T., Yla Herttuala, S., Yamamoto, R., Butler, S., Korpela, H., Salonen, R., et al. (1992) Autoantibody against oxidised LDL and progression of carotid atherosclerosis. *Lancet*, 339, 883–887.

[66] Palinski, W., Witztum, J.L. (2000) Immune responses to oxidative neoepitopes on LDL and phospholipids modulate the development of atherosclerosis. *J. Intern. Med*, 247, 371–380.

[67] Shaw, P.X., Horkko, S., Chang, M.K., Curtis, L.K., Palinski, W., et al. (2000) Natural antibodies with the T15 idiotype may act in atherosclerosis, apoptotic clearance, and protective immunity. *J. Clin. Invest*, 105, 1731–1734.

[68] Binder, C.J., Horkko, S., Dewan, A., Chang, M.K., Kieu, A.P., et al. (2003) Pneumococcal vaccination decreases atherosclerotic lesion formation: molecular mimicry between Streptococcus pneumoniae and oxidized LDL. *Nature Med*, 9, 736–743.

[69] Mehta, T.A., Greenman, J., Ettelaie, J., et al. (2005) Heat shock proteins in vascular disease--a review. *Eur. J. Vasc. Endovasc. Surg*, 29, 395–402.

[70] Lerman, A., Gibbons, R.J., Rodeheffer, R.J., Bailey KR, McKinley LJ, Heublein DM, Burnett JC Jr. (1993) Circulating N-terminal atrial natriuretic peptide as a marker for symptomless left-ventricular dysfunction. *Lancet*, 341, 1105-1109.

[71] Hoppichler, F., Lechleitner, M., Traweger, C., Schett G, Dzien A, Sturm W, Xu Q. (1996) Changes of serum antibodies to heat-shock protein 65 in coronary heart disease and acute myocardial infarction. *Atherosclerosis*, 126, 333–338.

[72] Hoshida, S., Nishino, M., Tanouchi, N., Kishimoto, T., Yamada, Y. (2005) Acute Chlamydia pneumoniae infection with heat-shock-protein-60-related response in patients with acute coronary syndrome. *Atherosclerosis*, 183, 109–212.

[73] Huittinen, T., Leinonen, M., Tenkanen, N., et al. (2002) Autoimmunity to human heat shock protein 60, Chlamydia pneumoniae infection, and inflammation in predicting coronary risk. *Arterioscler. Thromb Vasc. Biol*, 22, 431–437.

[74] Mayr, M., Metzler, B., Kiechl, S., Willeit, J., Schett, G., Xu, Q, Wick, G. (1999) Endothelial cytotoxicity mediated by serum antibodies to heat shock proteins of Escherichia coli and Chlamydia pneumoniae: immune reactions to heat shock proteins as a possible link between infection and atherosclerosis. *Circulation*, 99, 1560–1566.

[75] Andraws, R., Berger, J.S., Brown, D. (2005) Effects of antibiotic therapy on outcomes of patients with coronary artery disease: a meta-analysis of randomized controlled trials. *JAMA*, 293, 2641–2647.

[76] Ameli, S., Hultgardh-Nilsson, A., Regnström, J., Clara, F., Yano, J., Gercek, B., et al. (1996) Effect of immunization with homologous LDL and oxidized LDL on early atherosclerosis in hypercholesterolemic rabbits. *Arterioscler. Thromb Vasc. Biol*, 16, 1074–1079.

[77] Freigang, S., Hörkkö, S., Miller, E., Witztum, J. L., Palinski, W. (1998) Immunization of LDL receptor-deficient mice with homologous malondialdehyde-modified and native LDL reduces progression of atherosclerosis by mechanisms other than induction of high titers of antibodies to oxidative neoepitopes. *Arterioscler. Thromb Vasc. Biol*, 18, 1972–1982.

[78] Fredrikson, G.N., Soderberg, I., Lindholm, M., Dimayuga, P., Chyu, K.Y., Shah, P.K., Nilsson, J. (2003) Inhibition of atherosclerosis in apoE-null mice by immunization with apoB-100 peptide sequences. *Arterioscler. Thromb Vasc. Biol*, 23, 879–884.

[79] Afek, A., George, J., Gilburd, B., Rauova L, Goldberg I, Kopolovic J, Harats D, Shoenfeld Y. (2000) Immunization of low-density lipoprotein receptor deficient (LDL-RD) mice with heat shock protein 65 (HSP-65) promotes early atherosclerosis. *J. Autoimmun*, 14, 115–121.

[80] George, J., Afek, A., Gilburd, B., Blank M, Levy Y, Aron-Maor A, Levkovitz H, Shaish A, Goldberg I, Kopolovic J, Harats D, Shoenfeld Y. (1998) Induction of early atherosclerosis in LDL-receptor-deficient mice immunized with beta2-glycoprotein I. *Circulation*, 98, 1108–1115.

[81] Shoenfeld, Y., Harats, D., George, J. (1998) Atherosclerosis and the antiphospholipid syndrome: a link unravelled? *Lupus*, 7, 140–143.

[82] Matsuura, E., Kobayashi, K., Tabuchi, M., Lopes, L.R. (2006) Accelerated atheroma in the antiphospholipid syndrome. *Rheum. Dis. Clin. North Am*, 32, 537–551.

[83] George, J., Harats, D., Gilburd, B., Afek A, Shaish A, Kopolovic J, Shoenfeld Y. (2000) Adoptive transfer of beta(2)-glycoprotein I-reactive lymphocytes enhances early atherosclerosis in LDL receptor-deficient mice. *Circulation*, 102, 1822–1827.

[84] George, J., Afek, A., Gilburd, B., Levy Y, Blank M, Kopolovic J, Harats D, Shoenfeld Y. (1997) *Lupus*, 6, 723–729.

[85] Pereira I, Laurindo I, Burlingame R, Anjos L, Viana V, Leon E, Vendramini M, Borba E. (2008) Auto-antibodies do not influence development of atherosclerotic plaques in rheumatoid arthritis. *Joint Bone Spine*, 75, 416-421.

[86] Staub, H.L., Norman, G.L., Crowter, T., da Cunha, V.R., Polanczyk, A., Bohn, J.M., et al. (2003) Antibodies to the atherosclerotic plaque components beta2-glycoprotein I and heat-shock proteins as risk factors for acute cerebral ischemia. *Arq. Neuropsiquiatr*, 61, 757–763.

[87] Tedgui, A., Mallat, Z. (2006) Cytokines in atherosclerosis: pathogenic and regulatory pathways. *Physiol. Rev*, 86, 515–581.

[88] Mallat, Z., Besnard, S., Duriez, M., Deleuze V, Emmanuel F, Bureau MF, Soubrier F, Esposito B, Duez H, Fievet C, Staels B, Duverger N, Scherman D, Tedgui A. (1999) Protective role of interleukin-10 in atherosclerosis. *Circ. Res*, 85, e17–e24.

[89] Caligiuri, G., Rudling, M., Ollivier, V., Jacob, M.P., Michel, J.B., Hansson, G.K., Nicoletti, A. (2003) Interleukin-10 deficiency increases atherosclerosis, thrombosis, and low-density lipoproteins in apolipoprotein E knockout mice. *Mol. Med*, 9, 10–17.

[90] Gamble, J.R., Khew-Goodall, Y., Vadas, M.A. (1993) Transforming growth factor-beta inhibits E-selectin expression on human endothelial cells. *J. Immunol*, 150, 4494–4503.

[91] Argmann, C.A., Van Den Diepstraten, C.H., Sawyez, C.G., Edwards, J.Y., Hegele, R.A., Wolfe, B.M., et al. (2001) Transforming growth factor-beta1 inhibits macrophage cholesteryl ester accumulation induced by native and oxidized VLDL remnants. *Arterioscler. Thromb Vasc. Biol*, 21, 2011–2018.

[92] Virmani, R., Burke, A.P., Farb, A., et al. (2006) Pathology of the vulnerable plaque. *J. Am. Coll Cardiol*, 47, C13-C18.

[93] Thim, T., Hagensen, M.K., Bentzon, J.F., Falk, E. (2008) From vulnerable plaque to atherothrombosis. *J. Intern. Med*, 263, 506-516.

[94] Halvorsen, B., Otterdal, K., Dahl, T.B., Skjelland, M., Gullestad, L., Øie, E., Aukrust, P. (2008) Atherosclerotic plaque stability--what determines the fate of a plaque? *Prog. Cardiovasc. Dis*, 51, 183-194.

[95] Newby, A.C. (2007) Metalloproteinases and vulnerable atherosclerotic plaques. *Trends Cardiovasc. Med*, 17, 253-258.

[96] Libby, P., Sukhova, G., Lee, R.T., Galis ZS. (1995) Cytokines regulate vascular functions related to stability of the atherosclerotic plaque. *J. Cardiovasc. Pharmacol*, 25, 2, S9-S12.

[97] Kunte, H., Amberger, N., Busch, M.A., Rückert RI, Meiners S, Harms L. (2008) Markers of instability in high-risk carotid plaques are reduced by statins. *J. Vasc. Surg.* 47, 513-522.

[98] Galt, S.W., Lindemann, S., Allen, L., Medd, D.J., Falk, J.M., McIntyre, T.M., Prescott, S.M. (2002) Outside-in signals delivered by matrix metalloproteinase-1 regulate platelet function. *Circ. Res*, 90, 1093-1099.

[99] Sawicki, G., Sanders, E.J., Salas, E., Wozniak M, Rodrigo J, Radomski MW. (1998) Localization and translocation of MMP-2 during aggregation of human platelets. *Thromb Haemost*, 80, 836-839.

[100] Radomski, A., Stewart, M.W., Jurasz, P., Radomski, M.W. (2001) Pharmacological characteristics of solid-phase von Willebrand factor in human platelets. *Br. J. Pharmacol*, 134, 1013-1020.
[101] Lamaitre, V., O'Byrne, T.K., Borzcuk, A.C., et al. (2001) ApoE knockout mice expressing human matrix metalloproteinase-1 in macrophages have less advanced atherosclerosis. *J. Clin. Invest*, 107, 1227-1234.
[102] Kuzuya, M., Nakamura, K., Sasaki, T., et al. (2006) Effect of MMP-2 deficiency on atherosclerotic lesion formation in apoE-deficient mice. *Arterioscler. Thromb Vasc. Biol*, 26, 1120-1125.
[103] Galis, Z.S., Khatri, J.J. (2002) Matrix metalloproteinases in vascular remodeling and atherogenesis: the good, the bad, and the ugly. *Circ. Res*, 90, 251-262.
[104] Geng, Y.J., Libby, P. (2002) Progression of atheroma: a struggle between death and procreation. *Arterioscler. Thromb Vasc. Biol*, 22, 1370-1378.
[105] Littlewood, T.D., Bennett, M.R. (2003) Apoptotic cell death in atherosclerosis. *Curr. Opin. Lipidol*, 14, 469-476.
[106] Boyle, J.J., Weissberg, P.L., Bennett, M.R. (2003) Tumor necrosis factor-alpha promotes macrophage-induced vascular smooth muscle cell apoptosis by direct and autocrine mechanisms. *Arterioscler. Thromb Vasc. Biol*, 23, 1553-1558.
[107] Clarke, M.C., Figg, N., Maguire, J.J., Davenport AP, Goddard M, Littlewood TD, Bennett MR. (2006) Apoptosis of vascular smooth muscle cells induces features of plaque vulnerability in atherosclerosis. *Nat. Med*, 12, 1075-1080.
[108] Geng, Y.J., Libby, P. (1995) Evidence for apoptosis in advanced human atheroma. Colocalization with interleukin-1 beta-converting enzyme. *Am. J. Pathol*, 147, 251-266.
[109] Walsh, K., Smith, R.C., Kim, H.S. (2000) Vascular cell apoptosis in remodeling, restenosis, and plaque rupture. *Circ. Res*, 87, 184-188.
[110] Schaub, F.J., Han, D.K., Likes, W.C., et al. (2000) Fas/FADD-mediated activation of a specific program of inflammatory gene expression in vascular smooth muscle cells. *Nat. Med*, 6; 790-796.
[111] Tabas, I. (2005) Consequences and therapeutic implications of macrophage apoptosis in atherosclerosis: the importance of lesion stage and phagocytic efficiency. *Arterioscler. Thromb Vasc. Biol*, 25, 2255-2264.
[112] Halvorsen, B., Waehre, T., Scholz, H., Clausen OP, von der Thüsen JH, Müller F, Heimli H, Tonstad S, Hall C, Frøland SS, Biessen EA, Damås JK, Aukrust P. (2005) Interleukin-10 enhances the oxidized LDL-induced foam cell formation of macrophages by antiapoptotic mechanisms. *J. Lipid. Res*, 46, 211-219.
[113] Aukrust, P., Otterdal, K., Yndestad, A., Sandberg WJ, Smith C, Ueland T, Øie E, Damås JK, Gullestad L, Halvorsen B. (2008) The complex role of T-cell-based immunity in atherosclerosis. *Curr. Atheroscler. Rep*, 10, 236-243.
[114] Jeziorska, M., McCollum, C., Woolley, D.E. (1998) Calcification in atherosclerotic plaque of human carotid arteries: associations with mast cells and macrophages. *J. Pathol*, 185, 10-17.
[115] Di Girolamo, N., Wakefield, D. (2000) In vitro and in vivo expression of interstitial collagenase/MMP-1 by human mast cells. *Dev. Immunol*, 7, 131-142.
[116] Sun, J., Sukhova, G.K., Wolters, P.J., Yang M, Kitamoto S, Libby P, MacFarlane LA, Mallen-St Clair J, Shi GP. (2007) Mast cells promote atherosclerosis by releasing proinflammatory cytokines. *Nat. Med*, 13, 719-724.

[117] Li, N. (2008) Platelet-lymphocyte cross-talk. *J. Leukoc. Biol*, 83, 1069-1078.

[118] Damas, J.K., Otterdal, K., Yndestad, A., Aass H, Solum NO, Frøland SS, Simonsen S, Aukrust P, Andreassen AK. (2004) Soluble CD40 ligand in pulmonary arterial hypertension: possible pathogenic role of the interaction between platelets and endothelial cells. *Circulation*, 110, 999-1005.

[119] Weyrich, A., Cipollone, F., Mezzetti, A., Zimmerman, G. (2007) Platelets in atherothrombosis: new and evolving roles. *Curr. Pharm. Des*, 13, 1685-1691.

[120] Zarbock, A., Polanowska-Grabowska, R.K., Ley, K. (2007) Platelet-neutrophil-interactions: linking hemostasis and inflammation. *Blood Rev*, 21, 99-111.

[121] Weyrich, A.S., Elstad, M.R., McEver, R.P., McIntyre TM, Moore KL, Morrissey JH, Prescott SM, Zimmerman GA. (1996) Activated platelets signal chemokine synthesis by human monocytes. *J. Clin. Invest*, 97, 1525-1534.

[122] Waehre, T., Damas, J.K., Yndestad, A., Taskén K, Pedersen TM, Smith C, Halvorsen B, Frøland SS, Solum NO, Aukrust P. (2004) Effect of activated platelets on expression of cytokines in peripheral blood mononuclear cells - potential role of prostaglandin E2. *Thromb Haemost*, 92, 1358-1367.

[123] Kobashigawa, J. (2000) What is the optimal prophylaxis for treatment of cardiac allograft vasculopathy? *Curr. Control Trials Cardiovasc. Med*, 1, 166–171.

[124] Taylor, D.O., Edwards, L.B., Boucek, M.M., Trulock, E.P., Waltz, D.A., Keck, et al. (2006) Registry of the International Society for Heart and Lung Transplantation: twenty-third official adult heart transplantation report--2006. *J. Heart Lung Transplant*, 25, 869–879.

[125] Jimenez, J., Kapadia, S.R., Yamani, M.H., Platt L, Hobbs RE, Rincon G, Botts-Silverman C, Starling RC, Young JB, Nissen SE, Tuzcu M, Ratliff NB. (2001) Cellular rejection and rate of progression of transplant vasculopathy: a 3-year serial intravascular ultrasound study. *J. Heart Lung Transplant*, 20, 393–398.

[126] Hoang, K., Chen, Y.D., Reaven, G., Zhang, L., Ross, H., Billingham, M., et al. (1998) Diabetes and dyslipidemia. A new model for transplant coronary artery disease. *Circulation*, 97, 2160-2168.

[127] Vaziri ND. (2008) Mechanisms of lead-induced hypertension and cardiovascular disease. *Am. J. Physiol. Heart Circ. Physiol*, 295, H454-465.

[128] Johnson, D.E., Gao, S.Z., Schroeder, J.S., De-Campli, W.M., Billingham, M.E. (1989) The spectrum of coronary artery pathologic findings in human cardiac allografts. *J. Heart Lung Transplant*, 8, 349-359.

[129] Duquesnoy, R.J., Demetris, A.J. (1995) Immunopathology of cardiac transplant rejection. *Curr. Opin. Cardiol*, 10, 193-206.

[130] Rahmani, M., Cruz, R.P., Granville, D.J., McManus, B.M. (2006) Allograft vasculopathy versus atherosclerosis. *Circ. Res*, 99, 801-815.

[131] Costanzo, M.R., Naftel, D.C., Pritzker, M.R., Heilman, J.K., Boehmer, J.P,, Brozena, S.C., et al. (1998) Heart transplant coronary artery disease detected by coronary angiography: a multiinstitutional study of preoperative donor and recipient risk factors. Cardiac Transplant Research Database. *J. Heart Lung Transplant*, 17, 744-753.

[132] Uretsky, B.F., Murali, S., Reddy, G.S. (1987) Development of coronary artery disease in cardiac transplant patients receiving immunosuppressive therapy with cyclosporine and prednisone. *Circulation*, 76, 827-834.

[133] Schutz, A., KemKes, B.M., Kugler, C., Angermann, C., Schad, N., Rienmuller, R., Fritsch S, Anthuber M, Neumaier P, Gokel JM. (1990) The influence of rejection episodes on the development of coronary artery disease after heart transplantation. *Eur. J. Cardiothorac. Surg*, 4, 300-307.

[134] Forbes, R.D., Zheng, S.X., Gommersall, M., Gutmann, R.D. (1997) Irreversible chronic vascular rejection occurs only after development of advanced allograft vasculopathy: a comparative study of a rat cardiac allograft model using a retransplantation protocol. *Transplantation*, 63, 743–749.

[135] Berg KK, Madsen HO, Garred P, Wiseth R, Gunnes S, Videm V. (2009) The additive contribution from inflammatory genetic markers on the severity of cardiovascular disease. *Scand. J. Immunol*, 69, 36-42.

[136] Hosenpud, J.D., Everett, J.P., Morris, T.E., Mauck KA, Shipley GD, Wagner CR. (1995) Cardiac allograft vasculopathy. Association with cell-mediated but not humoral alloimmunity to donor-specific vascular endothelium. *Cirulation*, 92, 205–211.

[137] Hruban, R.H., Beschorner, W.E., Baumgarther, W.A., Augustine SM, Ren H, Reitz BA, Hutchins GM. (1990) Accelerated arteriosclerosis in heart transplant recipients is associated with a T-lymphocyte-mediated endothelialitis. *Am. J. Pathol*, 137,871–882.

[138] Page, C., Rose, M., Yacoub, M., Pigott, R. (1992) Antigenic heterogeneity of vascular endothelium. *Am. J. Pathol*, 141, 673–683.

[139] Taylor, P.M., Rose, M.L., Yacoub, M.H. (1993) Coronary artery immunogenicity: a comparison between explanted recipient or donor hearts and transplanted hearts. *Transpl. Immunol*, 1, 294–301.

[140] Rogers, N.J., Lechler, R.I. (2001) Allorecognition. *Am. J. Transplant*, 1, 97–102.

[141] Lechler, R., Ng, W.F., Steinman, R.M. (2001) Dendritic cells in transplantation--friend or foe? *Immunity*, 14, 357–368.

[142] Smyth, L.A., Herrera, O.B., Golshayan,D., Lombardi, G., Lechler, R.I. (2006) A novel pathway of antigen presentation by dendritic and endothelial cells: Implications for allorecognition and infectious diseases. *Transplantation*, 82, S15–S18.

[143] Fischbein, M.P., Yun, J., Laks, H., Irie, Y., Fishbein, M.C., Espejo, M., et al. (2001) CD8+ lymphocytes augment chronic rejection in a MHC class II mismatched model. *Transplantation*, 71, 1146-1153.

[144] Szeto, W.Y., Krasinskas, A.M., Kreisel, D., Krupnick, A.S., Popma, S.H., Rosengard, B.R. (2002) Depletion of recipient CD4+ but not CD8+ T lymphocytes prevents the development of cardiac allograft vasculopathy. *Transplantation*, 73, 1116-1122.

[145] Choi, J., Enis, D.R., Koh, K.P., Shiao, S.L., Pober, J.S. (2004) T lymphocyte-endothelial cell interactions. *Annu. Rev. Immunol*, 22, 683–709.

[146] Salomon, R.N., Hughes, C.C., Schoen, F.J., Payne DD, Pober JS, Libby P. (1991) Human coronary transplantation-associated arteriosclerosis. Evidence for a chronic immune reaction to activated graft endothelial cells. *Am. J. Pathol*, 138, 791–798.

[147] Hosenpud, J.D., Edwards, E.B., Lin, H.M., Daily, P. (1996) Influence of HLA matching on thoracic transplant outcomes. An analysis from the UNOS/ISHLT Thoracic Registry. *Circulation*, 94, 170 –174.

[148] Kaczmarek, I., Deutsch, M.A., Rohrer, M.E., Beiras-Fernandez, A., Groetzner, J., Daebritz, S., et al. (2006) HLA-DR matching improves survival after heart transplantation: is it time to change allocation policies? *J. Heart Lung Transplant*, 25, 1057–1062.

[149] Holvoet, P., Stassen, J.M., Van Jleemput, J., et al. (1998) Oxidized low density lipoproteins in patients with transplant-associated coronary artery disease. *Arterioscler. Thromb Vasc. Biol*, 18, 100–107.

[150] Ardehali, A., Laks, H., Drinkwater, D.C., Ziv, E., Drake, T.A. (1995) Vascular cell adhesion molecule-1 is induced on vascular endothelia and medial smooth muscle cells in experimental cardiac allograft vasculopathy. *Circulation*, 92, 450-456.

[151] Labarrere, C.A., Pitts, D., Nelson, D.R., Faulk, W.P. (1995) Coronary artery disease in cardiac allografts: association with arteriolar endothelial HLA-DR and ICAM-1 antigens. *Transplant Proc*, 27, 1939-1940.

[152] Ravalli, S., Szabolcs, M., Albala, A., Michler, R.E., Cannon, P.J. (1996) Increased immunoreactive endothelin-1 in human transplant coronary artery disease. *Circulation*, 94, 2096–2102.

[153] Weis, M., Cooke, J.P. (2003) Cardiac allograft vasculopathy and dysregulation of the NO synthase pathway. *Arterioscler. Thromb. Vasc. Biol.*, 23, 567–575.

[154] Zhang, J., Patel, J.M., Li, Y.D., Block, E.R. (1997) Proinflammatory cytokines downregulate gene expression and activity of constitutive nitric oxide synthase in porcine pulmonary artery endothelial cells. *Res. Commun. Mol. Pathol. Pharmacol*, 96, 71–87.

[155] Ito, A., Tsao, P.S., Adimoolam, S., Kimoto, M., Ogawa, T., Cooke, J.P. (1999) Novel mechanism for endothelial dysfunction: dysregulation of dimethylarginine dimethylaminohydrolase. *Circulation*, 99, 3092–3095.

[156] Taylor, D.O., Edwards, L.B., Boucek, M.M., Trulock, E.P., Aurora, P., Christie J., et. al. (2007) Registry of the International Society for Heart and Lung Transplantation: twenty-fourth official adult heart transplant report--2007. *J. Heart Lung Transplant*, 26, 769-781.

[157] Ma, H.,. Calderon, T.M., Fallon, J.T., Berman, J.W. (2002) Hepatocyte growth factor is a survival factor for endothelial cells and is expressed in human atherosclerotic plaques. *Atherosclerosis*, 164, 79-87.

[158] Turka, L.A., Linsley, P.S., Lin, H., Brady, W., Leiden, J.M., Wei, R.Q., et al. (1992) T-cell activation by the CD28 ligand B7 is required for cardiac allograft rejection in vivo. *Proc. Natl. Acad. Sci. USA*, 89, 11102-11105.

[159] Savage, C.O.S., Hughs, C.C.C.W., McIntyre, B.W., Picard, J.K., Pober, J.S. (1993) Human CD4+ T cells proliferate to HLA-DR+ allogeneic vascular endothelium. Identification of accessory interactions. *Transplantation*, 56, 128-134.

[160] Rabinovitch, M,. Molossi, S., Clausell, N. (1995) Cytokine-mediated fibronectin production and transendothelial migration of lymphocytes in the mechanism of cardiac allograft vascular disease: efficacy of novel therapeutic approaches. *J. Heart Lung Transplant*, 14, S116-S123.

[161] Chai S, Chai Q, Danielsen CC, Hjorth P, Nyengaard JR, Ledet T, Yamaguchi Y, Rasmussen LM, Wogensen L. (2005) Overexpression of hyaluronan in the tunica media promotes the development of atherosclerosis. *Circ. Res*, 96, 83-91.

[162] Gibbons, G.H. (1995) The pathogenesis of graft vascular disease: implications of vascular remodeling. *J. Heart Lung Transplant*, 14, S149-S158.

[163] Pinto, .F.J, Chenzbraun, A., Botas, J., Valantine, H.A., St Goar, F.G., Alderman, E.L. et al. (1994) Feasibility of serial intracoronary ultrasound imaging for assessment of

progression of intimal proliferation in cardiac transplant recipients. *Circulation*, 90, 2348-2355.

[164] von Scheidt, W., Erdmann, E. (1991) Dilated angiopathy: a specific subtype of allograft coronary artery disease. *J. Heart Lung Transplant*, 10, 698-703.

[165] Michaels, P.J., Espejo, M.L., Kobashigawa, J., Alejos JC, Burch C, Takemoto S, Reed EF, Fishbein MC. (2003) Humoral rejection in cardiac transplantation: risk factors, hemodynamic consequences and relationship to transplant coronary artery disease. *J. Heart Lung Transplant*, 22, 58-69.

[166] Fredrich, R., Toyoda, M, Czer, R.S., Galfayan K, Galera O, Trento A, Freimark D, Young S, Jordan SC. (1999) The clinical significance of antibodies to human vascular endothelial cells after cardiac transplantation. *Transplantation*, 67, 385–391.

[167] Dunn, M.J., Crisp, S.J., Rose, M.L., Taylor, P.M., Yacoub, M.H. (1992) Anti-endothelial antibodies and coronary artery disease after cardiac transplantation. *Lancet*, 339, 1566–1570.

[168] Wheeler, C.H., Collins, A., Dunn, M.J., Crisp, S.J., Yacoub, M.H., Rose, M.L. (1995) Characterization of endothelial antigens associated with transplant-associated coronary artery disease. *J. Heart Lung Transplant*, 14, S188–S197.

[169] Wu GW, Kobashigawa JA, Fishbein MC, Patel JK, Kittleson MM, Reed EF, Kiyosaki KK, Ardehali A. (2009) Asymptomatic antibody-mediated rejection after heart transplantation predicts poor outcomes. *J. Heart Lung Transplant*, 28, 417-422.

[170] Terasaki, P.I. (2003) Humoral theory of transplantation. *Am. J. Transplant*, 3, 665-673.

[171] Reed, E.F., Demetris, A.J., Hammond, E., Itescu S, Kobashigawa JA, Reinsmoen NL, Rodriguez ER, Rose M, Stewart S, Suciu-Foca N, Zeevi A, Fishbein MC; International Society for Heart and Lung Transplantation. (2006) Acute antibody-mediated rejection of cardiac transplants. *J. Heart Lung Transplant*, 25,153-159.

[172] Hammond, E.H., Yowell, R.L., Price, G.D., Menlove, R.L., Olsen, S.L., O'Connell, J.B., Bristow, M.R., Doty, D.B., Millar, R.C., Karwande, S.V., et al. (1992) Vascular rejection and its relationship to allograft coronary artery disease. *J. Heart Lung Transplant*, 11, S111-S119.

[173] Rose, E.A., Pepino, P., Barr, M.L., Smith, J.R., Ratner, A.J., Ho, E., Berger, C. (1992) Relation of HLA antibodies and graft atherosclerosis in human cardiac allograft recipients. *J. Heart Lung Transplant*, 11, S120–S123.

[174] Takemoto, S.K., Zeevi, A., Feng, S., Colvin, R.B., Jordan, S., Kobashigawa, J., Kupiec-Weglinski, J., Matas, A., Montgomery, R.A., Nickerson, P., Platt, J.L., Rabb, H., Thistlethwaite, R., Tyan, D., Delmonico, F.L. (2004) National conference to assess antibody-mediated rejection in solid organ transplantation. *Am. J. Transplant*, 4, 1033-1041.

[175] Kaczmarek, I., Deutsch, M.A., Kauke, T., Beiras-Fernandez, A., Schmoeckel, M., Vicol, C., Sodian, R., Reichart, B., Spannagl, M., Ueberfuhr, P. (2008) Donor-specific HLA alloantibodies: long-term impact on cardiac allograft vasculopathy and mortality after heart transplant. *Exp. Clin. Transplant*, 6, 229-235.

[176] Colvin, R.B., Smith, R.N. (2005) Antibody-mediated organ-allograft rejection. *Nat. Rev. Immunol*, 5, 807-817.

[177] Wehner, J., Morrell, C.N., Reynolds, T., Rodriguez, E.R., Baldwin, W.M. (2007) Antibody and complement in transplant vasculopathy. *Circ. Res*, 100, 191-203.

[178] Sims, P.J., Wiedmer, T. (1991) The response of human platelets to activated components of the complement system. *Immunol. Today*, 12, 338–340.

[179] Sims, P.J., Wiedmer, T. (1995) Induction of cellular procoagulant activity by the membrane attack complex of complement. *Semin. Cell Biol*, 6, 275–282.

[180] Hattori, R., Hamilton, K.K., McEver, R.P., Sims, P.J. (1989) Complement proteins C5b-9 induce secretion of high molecular weight multimers of endothelial von Willebrand factor and translocation of granule membrane protein GMP-140 to the cell surface. *J. Biol. Chem*, 264, 9053-9060.

[181] Saadi, S., Holzknecht, R.A., Patte, C.P., Stern, D.M., Platt, J.L. (1995) Complement-mediated regulation of tissue factor activity in endothelium. *J. Exp. Med*, 182, 1807–1814.

[182] Johnson, E., Hetland, G. (1991) Human umbilical vein endothelial cells synthesize functional C3, C5, C6, C8 and C9 in vitro. *Scand. J. Immunol*, 33, 667–671.

[183] Ramm, L.E., Whitlow, M.B., Koski, C.L., Shin, M.L., Mayer, M.M. (1983) Elimination of complement channels from the plasma membranes of U937, a nucleated mammalian cell line: temperature dependence of the elimination rate. *J. Immunol.* 131, 1411–1415.

[184] Baldwin, W.M. 3rd, Pruitt, S.K., Brauer, R.B., Daha, M.R., (1995) Complement in organ transplantation. Contributions to inflammation, injury and rejection. *Transplantation*, 59, 797-808.

[185] Andrade, C.F., Waddell, T.K., Keshavjee, S., Liu, M. (2005) Innate immunity and organ transplantation: the potential role of toll-like receptors. *Am. J. Transplant*, 5, 969 –975.

[186] Obhrai, J., Goldstein, D.R. (2006) The role of toll-like receptors in solid organ transplantation. *Transplantation*, 81, 497–502.

[187] Methe, H., Zimmer, E., Grimm, C., Nabauer, M., Koglin, J. (2004) Evidence for a role of toll-like receptor 4 in development of chronic allograft rejection after cardiac transplantation. *Transplantation*, 78, 1324 –1331.

[188] Gohra, H., MacDonal, T.O., Verrier, E.D., Aziz, S. (1995) Endothelial loss and regeneration in a model of transplant arteriosclerosis. *Transplantation*, 60, 96-102.

[189] Minami, E., Laflamme, M.A,. Saffitz, J.E., Murry, C.E. (2005) Extracardiac progenitor cells repopulate most major cell types in the transplanted human heart. *Circulation*, 112, 2951–2958.

[190] Simper, D., Wang, S., Deb, A., Holmes, D., McGregor, C., Frantz, R., Kushwaha, S.S., et. al. (2003) Endothelial progenitor cells are decreased in blood of cardiac allograft patients with vasculopathy and endothelial cells of noncardiac origin are enriched in transplant atherosclerosis. *Circulation*, 108, 143–149.

[191] Dong, C., Redenbach, D., Wood, S., Battistini, B., Wilson, J.E., McManus, B.M. (1996) The pathogenesis of cardiac allograft vasculopathy. *Curr. Opin. Cardiol*, 11, 183-190.

[192] Kaczmarek, I., Ertl, B., Scmauss, D., et al. (2006) Preventing cardiac allograft vasculopathy: long-term beneficial effects of mycophenolate mofetil. *J. Heart Lung Transplant*, 25, 550-556.

[193] Keogh, A., Richardson, M., Ruygrok, P., et al. (2004) Sirolimus in de novo heart transplant recipients reduces acute rejection and prevents coronary artery disease at 2 years: a randomized clinical trial. *Circulation*, 110, 2694-2700.

[194] Guilherme, L., Fae, K.C., Oshiro, S.C., et al. (2007) T cell response in rheumatic fever: crossreactivity between streptococcal M protein peptides and heart tissue proteins. *Curr. Protein Pept. Sci*, 8, 39-44.
[195] Guilherme, L., Fae, K., Oshiro, S.C., Kalil, J. (2005) Molecular pathogenesis of rheumatic fever and rheumatic heart disease. *Expert Rev. Mol. Med*, 7, 1-15.
[196] Guilherme, L., Fae, K., Oshiro, et al. (2005) Rheumatic fever: how S. pyogenes-primed peripheral T cells trigger heart valve lesions. *Ann. N. Y. Acad. Sci*, 1051, 132-140.
[197] Gorton, D., Govan, B., Olive, C., Ketheesan, N. (2009) B- and T-cell responses in group a streptococcus M-protein- or Peptide-induced experimental carditis. *Infect Immun*, 77, 2177-2183.
[198] Dale, J.B., Beachey, E.H. (1985) Epitopes of streptococcal M proteins shared with cardiac myosin. *J. Exp. Med*, 162, 583-591.
[199] Cunningham, M.W. (2000) Pathogenesis of group A streptococcal infections. *Clin. Microbiol. Rev*, 13, 470–511.
[200] Cunningham M.W. (2004) T cell mimicry in inflammatory heart disease. *Mol. Immunol*, 40, 1121-1127.
[201] Galvin, J.E., Hemric, M.E., Ward, K. Cunningham, M.W. (2000) Cytotoxic mAb from rheumatic carditis recognizes heart valves and laminin. *J. Clin. Invest*, 106, 217-224.
[202] Guilherme, L., Ramasawmy, R., Kalil, J. (2007) Rheumatic fever and rheumatic heart disease: genetics and pathogenesis. *Scand. J. Immun*, 66, 199–207.
[203] Morris, K., Mohan, C., Wahi, P.L., et al. (1993) Enhancement of IL-1, IL-2 production and IL-2 receptor generation in patients with acute rheumatic fever and active rheumatic heart disease; a prospective study. *Clin. Exp. Immunol*, 91, 429-436.
[204] Guilherme, L., Curry, P., Demarchi, L.M., et al. (2004) Rheumatic heart disease: proinflammatory cytokines play a role in the progression and maintenance of valvular lesions. *Am. J. Pathol*, 165, 1583-1591.
[205] Soderstrom, T., Soderstrom, R., Enskog, A. (1991) Immunoglobulin subclasses and prophylactic use of immunoglobulin in immunoglobulin G subclass deficiency. *Cancer*, 68, 1426.
[206] Cox, J.S., Chen, B., McNeil, M., Jacobs, W.R., Jr. (1999) Complex lipid determines tissue-specific replication of Mycobacterium tuberculosis in mice. *Nature*, 402, 79-83.
[207] Ludwiczak, P., Gilleron, M., Bordat, Y., et al. (2002) Mycobacterium tuberculosis phoP mutant: lipoarabinomannan molecular structure. *Microbiology*, 148, 3029.
[208] Sara, S.K., 2006, Uludag Üniversitesi Tıp Fakültesi Ders Notları.
[209] Prigozy, T.I., Sieling, P.A., Clemens, D., et al. (1997) The mannose receptor delivers lipoglycan antigens to endosomes for presentation to T cells by CD1b molecules. *Immunity*, 6, 187-197.
[210] Bozdoğan, G., Doğu F., Ikinciogulları A., Babacan E. (2004) *Turkiye Klinikleri J. Pediatr*, 13, 238.
[211] Lutskiy, M.I., Park, J.Y., Remold, S.K., Remold-O'Donnell, E. (2008) Evolution of highly polymorphic T cell populations in siblings with the Wiskott-Aldrich Syndrome. *PloS One*, 3, e3444.
[212] Barnett, D., Walker, B., Landay, A., Denny, T.N. (2008) CD4 immunophenotyping in HIV infection. *Nat. Rev. Microbiol*, 6, S7-S15.

[213] Hogg, J.C., Chu, F., Utokaparch, S., Woods, R., Elliott, W.M., Buzatu, L., et al. (2004) The nature of small-airway obstruction in chronic obstructive pulmonary disease. *N. Engl. J. Med*, 350, 2645-2653.

[214] Di Stefano, A., Caramori, G., Gnemmi, I., Contoli, M., Vicari, C., Capelli, A., Magno, F., D'Anna, S.E., Zanini, A., Brun, P., Casolari, P., Chung, K.F., Barnes, P.J., Papi, A., Adcock, I., Balbi, B. (2009) T helper type 17-related cytokine expression is increased in the bronchial mucosa of stable chronic obstructive pulmonary disease patients. *Clin. Exp. Immunol*, 157, 316-324.

[215] Wynn, T.A. (2003) IL-13 effector functions. *Annu. Rev. Immunol*, 21, 425-456.

[216] Elias, J.A., Lee, C.G., Zheng, T., Shim, Y., Zhu, Z. (2003) Interleukin-13 and leukotrienes: an intersection of pathogenetic schema. *Am. J. Respir. Cell Mol. Biol*, 28, 401-404.

[217] Mattes, J., et al. (2001) IL-13 induces airways hyperreactivity independently of the IL-4R alpha chain in the allergic lung. *J. Immunol*, 167, 1683-1692.

[218] Grunewald, J., Eklund, A. (2007) Role of CD4+ T cells in sarcoidosis. *Proc. Am. Thorac. Soc*, 15, 4, 461-464.

[219] Laberge, M.A., Moore, K.J., Freeman, M.W. (2005) Atherosclerosis and innate immune signaling. *Ann. Med.*, 37(2), 130-40.

[220] Nilsson, J., Hansson, G.K. (2008) Autoimmunity in atherosclerosis: a protective response loosing control? *J. Int. Med.*, 263(5), 464-78.

[221] Yan, Z., Hansson, G.K. (2007) Innate immunity, macrophage activation, and atherosclerosis. *Immunol. Rev.*, 219(1), 187-203.

[222] Segers, D., Garcia-Garcia, H.M., Cheng, C., de Crom, R., Krams, R., Wentzel, J.J., van der Steen, A.F., Serruys, P.W., Leenen, P.J., Laman, J.D. 2008 A primer on the immune system in the pathogenesis and treatment of atherosclerosis. *EuroIntervention*, 4, 378-390.

[223] Schmauss, D., Weis, M. 2008 Cardiac allograft vasculopathy: recent developments. *Circulation*, 117, 2131-2141.

In: Immunology in Clinic Practice
Editor: Cagatay Oktenli, pp. 77-83

ISBN 978-1-60876-644-4


*Chapter 5*

# OVERVIEW OF RECENT IMMUNOLOGICAL RESEARCH IN OPHTHALMOLOGY

***Ali Hakan Durukan and Tarkan Mumcuoğlu***
Department of Ophthalmology,
Gülhane Military Medical Academy, Ankara, Turkey

## ABSTRACT

The eye is a common target of inflammatory responses included by local and systemic immunologic reactions; therefore it is vulnerable to a variety of immunologically mediated diseases. Since the transparency of the visual axis is absolutely required for accurate vision, the eye can tolerate inflammation to only a very limited degree. The conventional type of immunity generated while antigens or pathogens penetrating through the skin has almost never been observed in the normal eye. Accordingly, any immune responses taking place in or on the eye are regulated. The eye is immunologically unique because it has no formed lymph nodes. On the ocular surface, immunity reactions resemble those observed on the other mucosal surfaces. As the evidence has still been accumulating the effect of inflammatory events in the pathogenesis of age-related macular degeneration, a new idea has been suggested that anti-inflammatory drugs might postpone the degeneration process.

**Keywords:** eye; ocular surface immunity; conjunctival surface; glaucoma; sclera; retina; macular degeneration

## INTRODUCTION

It is an inevitable fact that all tissues have the need for immune protection from invading or endogenous pathogens. Immune system exists in harmony with a variety of immune effectors, since pathogens with different virulence strategies impend different types of tissues. Immune system can act in turn to a specific pathogen or antigen in a particular tissue effective in eliminating the threat and simultaneously will not damage the tissue itself. Different tissues and organs display markedly different susceptibility to immune-mediated tissue injury [1].

The eye is a common target of inflammatory response and it is vulnerable to a variety of immunologically mediated diseases. Because the transparency of the visual axis is absolutely required for accurate vision, the eye can tolerate inflammation to only a very limited degree. The conventional type of immunity while antigens or pathogens penetrating through the skin has almost never been observed in the normal eye. Accordingly, any immune responses taking place in or on the eye are regulated [1].

Four layers of the eye are commonly involved in immunologic reactions:

a. Tear fluid layer and conjunctiva; The anterior portion of the eye and provides the primary barrier against infectious patogens, aeroallergens, and chemical substances
b. The sclera; collagenous and basically involved in connective tissue diseases
c. The uvea; highly vascular part and principally affected in inflammatory disorders associated with cell-mediated hypersensitivity reactions and circulating immune complexes
d. The retina; practically an extension of the central nervous system.

The eye is immunologically unique because it has no formed lymph nodes. On the ocular surface, immunity resembles that observed on other mucosal surfaces. Within the eye, an unusual form of immunity is observed.

## Ocular Surface Immunity

The conjunctiva is the most immunologically active tissue of the external eye and it is an active participant in immune defense of the ocular surface against invasion by exogenous substances. In this way, it undergoes lymphoid hyperplasia in response to a stimulant [2]. Histologically, the conjunctiva has two layers: the epithelial and substansia propria layers. Inflammatory cells (eosinophils, basophils or mast cells) are commonly found in the layer just below the epithelial surface.

The conjunctival surface is immersed with a thin layer of tear film which is orderly comprised of an outer lipid layer, a middle aqueous layer which contains a variety of solutes (immunologically active proteins, enzymes, carbohydrates, electrolytes), and an inner mucoprotein layer. Immune cells are transported by blood vessels and lymphatic channels. Dendritic cells, T and B lymphocytes, mast cells, and neutrophils are major immune cells found in regular human conjunctiva. Dendritic cells act as antigen-presenting cells to T lymphocytes and may stimulate antigen-specific class II region-mediated T-lymphocyte proliferation [3]. T-lymphocytes are the prevailing lymphocyte subpopulation in conjunctiva and act as the main effector cells in immune reactions such as delayed hypersensitivity or cytotoxic responses. B lymphocytes are absent in conjuctiva. On the other hand, plasma cells are detected only in the conjunctival accessory lacrimal glands of Krause or in minor lacrimal glands [4]. T and B lymphocytes and plasma cells are also present between the acini of the major lacrimal gland. Plasma cells from major and minor lacrimal glands synthesize immunoglobulins, mainly IgA [5,6], which is released to the luminal surface of the ducts associated with a secretory component and discharged with the tear film. Secretory IgA is a protectant of mucosal surfaces.

Neutrophils and macrophages are aided to destroy antigens by immunoglobulins and lymphokines generated of the lymphoid tissue of the conjunctiva. The arrival of neutrophils and macrophages is facilitated by mast cells and complement.

The unique anatomic and physiologic peculiarity of the human cornea explain its predilection for involvement in diversified immune disorders and its ability to express immune privilege. The peripheral cornea is closer to the conjunctiva in which blood vessels and lymphatic channels make a mechanism available for the afferent arc of corneal immune reactions. Blood vessels derived from the anterior conjunctival and deep episcleral arteries extend 0.5 mm into the clear cornea [7]. This situation makes the peripheral cornea more susceptible than the central cornea to involvement in a wide variety of autoimmune and hypersensitive disorders.

The sclera consists almost entirely of collagen and proteogylcans. Normal human sclera has few if any lymphocytes, macrophages, Langerhans' cells, or neutrophils [8]. In the sclera, the cells flow past briskly from blood vessels of the episclera and choroid reacting to an inflammatory stimulus. Because of the collagenous nature of the sclera, many systemic autoimmune disorders may affect it [8,9].

### Intraocular Immunology

Madewar and associates [10] investigated immune privileged sites and they recognized extended survival of foreign tissue grafts placed in the eye or in the brain. They also postulated that immune privilege resulted from immunologic ignorance [10]. It represents the most extreme form of the concept of regional immunity. In the normal eye, immune privileged sites are subretinal space, vitreal cavity, and anterior chamber.

The aqueous humor contributes to this local ocular defense system [11]. The anterior chamber of the eye shows resistance to inflammation [12] and works as an antigen depot [13]. The forces to shape immune privilege include microanatomic, biomechanic, and immuneregulatory characteristics. Passive features such as blood-ocular barrier, lack of lymphatics, and low expression of major histocompatibility complex class I and class II molecules are important for immune privilege. Besides, immunomodulatory molecules expressed on ocular tissues and present in ocular fluids have active role in privilege.

## Immunologic Factors in the Pathogenesis of Glaucoma

Glaucoma is a chronic neurodegenerative disease characterized by optic nerve degeneration and progressive loss of retinal ganglion cells and their axons [14,15]. Elevated intraocular pressure is considered a major, but not sole risk factor, and treatment to reduce intraocular pressure does not always prevent progression of the disease [16,17]. Another factors such as apoptotis [18], increased nitric oxide levels [19], and autoimmunity [20] are also proposed. Retinal ganglion cell death is thought to occur by an apoptotic mechanism triggered by multiple mechanisms [21]. Normally, activated T cells are able to enter the central nervous system as a part of immune surveillance [22,23]. In glaucoma, the protective immunity has been suggested to minimize injury to the optic nerve by reducing the secondary degeneration of neurons [24].

In normal tension glaucoma, Wax et al. reported increased antibody reactivity and heat shock protein (HSP) 60 antibodies [25,26]. They proposed that this may indicate a generalized response to tissue stress or damage [26]. Then, higher levels of antibodies against small HSPs were also detected in glaucoma patients [27]. The authors suggested that direct application of these antibodies on isolated human retina results in apoptosis of neurons [27]. In human donor eyes with glaucoma, increased HSP27 and HSP60 expression were reported in retina and optic nerve head [28].

Antibodies are able to modulate the activity of target molecules and influence their physiologic functions [29-33]. On the other hand, up-regulated antibodies are explained as an initiation of autoagressive sequences [34,35]. In glaucoma, it was hypothesized that the loss of some protective autoantibodies may lead to a loss of immune protection [36].

## Immune Mechanisms in the Pathogenesis of Age-Related Macular Degeneration

Age-related macular degeneration (AMD) is the leading cause of blindness in individuals 65 years of age and over in industrialized world [37,38]. Although the causes of AMD are currently unknown, immunological factors may play a role in the pathogenesis of AMD [39]. Inflammatory cells such as T cells, mast cells and macrophages have been suggested in histopathologic evaluation of AMD lesions [40].

Drusen are considered important risk factors in the pathogenesis of AMD. Drusen are characterized as extracellular deposits situated between the RPE cell layer and Bruch's membrane [41]. Moreover, these deposits may cause an inflammatory event leading to further depositions [39]. Anderson et al. reported that drusens have C-reactive protein and components of complement in their cytoplasm [41]. RPE cells have been shown to express the receptor for C5a [42].

In a few studies, it has been proposed that the autoimmunity might play a role in the pathogenesis of AMD [43, 44]. As the evidence is still accumulating about the effect of inflammatory events in the pathogenesis of AMD, a new idea has been suggested that anti-inflammatory drugs might postpone the degeneration process. However, it has been suggested that there is no association between the use of systemic anti-inflammatory drugs and either the cross-sectional prevalence or the longitudinal incidence of AMD [45].

## Conclusion

Immunology of the eye evolved during the last century as a subspecialty linking immunologists and ophthalmologists [46]. In this way, this subspecialty may provide new treatment alternatives in ophthalmological diseases [46].

Immunotherapy for AMD is a new method [47,48]. It has been recently reported another technique whereby the CNV is selectively targeted via chimeric antibodies [49]. Treatment of animals with this chimeric antibody prevented the formation of laser induced choroidal neovascularization.

## REFERENCES

[1] Streilen, J.W. (1997) Regional immunology of the eye, Pepose, JW., Holland, G.N., Wilhemus, K.R. (Ed.), Ocular Infection and Immunity, Mosby, Philadelphia, 19.

[2] Steven, P., Gebert, A. (2009) Conjunctiva-associated lymphoid tissue - current knowledge, animal models and experimental prospects. *Ophthalmic Res*, 42, 2-8.

[3] Shoji, J., Inada, N., Saito, K., Takaura, N., Iwasaki, Y., Sawa, M. (1998) Immunohistochemical study on follicular dendritic cell of conjunctiva-associated lymphoid tissue. *Jpn. J. Ophthalmol*, 42, 1-7.

[4] Sacks, E., Wieczorek, R., Jacobiec, F.A., et al. (1986) Lymphocytic subpopulations in the normal human conjunctiva. A monoclonal antibody study. *Ophthalmology*, 93, 1279.

[5] Knop, E., Knop, N., Claus, P. (2008) Local production of secretory IgA in the eye-associated lymphoid tissue (EALT) of the normal human ocular surface. *Invest Ophthalmol. Vis. Sci*, 49, 2322-2329.

[6] Wieczorek, R., Jacobiec, F.A., Sacks, E., Knowles, D.M. (1988) The immunoarchitecture of the normal human lacrimal gland. Relevancy for understanding pathologic conditions. *Ophthalmology*, 95, 100-109.

[7] Hogan, M.J., Alvarado, J.A., Weddell, J.E. (1971) Histology of the Human Eye: An Atlas and Textbook, W.B. Saunders, Philadelphia, 112.

[8] Fong, L.P., Sainz de la Maza, M., Rice, B.A., Kupferman, A.E., Foster, C.S. (1991) Immunopathology of scleritis. *Ophthalmology*, 98, 472-479.

[9] Watson, P.G., Young, R.D. (2004) Scleral structure, organisation and disease. A review. *Exp. Eye Res*, 78, 609-623.

[10] Madewar, P.B. (1961) Immunological tolerance. *Science*, 133, 303.

[11] Taylor, A.W., Streilein, J.W., Cousins, S.W. (1992) Identification of alpha-melanocyte stimulating hormone as a potential immunosuppressive factor in aqueous humor. *Curr. Eye Res*, 11, 1199-1206.

[12] Cousins, S.W., Trattler, W.B., Streilein, J.W. (1991) Immune privilege and suppression of immunogenic inflammation in the anterior chamber of the eye. *Curr. Eye Res*, 10, 287-297.

[13] Wilbanks, G.A., Streilein, J.W. (1989) The differing patterns of antigen release and local retention following anterior chamber and intravenous inoculation of soluble antigen. Evidence that the eye acts as an antigen depot. *Reg. Immunol*, 2, 390-398.

[14] Quigley, H.A. (1993) Open-angle glaucoma. *N. Engl. J. Med*, 328, 1097-1106.

[15] Quigley, H.A. (1996) Number of people with glaucoma worldwide. *Br. J. Ophthalmol*, 80, 389-393.

[16] Tezel, G., Siegmund, K.D., Trinkaus, K., et al. (2001) Clinical factors associated with progression of glaucomatous optic disc damage in treated patients. *Arch Ophthalmol*, 119, 813-818.

[17] Society TEG. (2006) Terminology and guidelines for glaucoma, 2nd ed.

[18] Vrabec, J.P., Levin, L.A. (2007) The neurobiology of cell death in glaucoma. *Eye*, 21 Suppl 1, S11-14.

[19] Neufeld, A.H., Hernandez, M.R., Gonzalez, M. (1997) Nitric oxide synthase in the human glaucomatous optic nerve head. *Arch. Ophthalmol*, 115, 497-503.

[20] Wax, M.B. (2000) Is there a role for the immune system in glaucomatous optic neuropathy? *Curr. Opin. Ophthalmol*, 11, 145-150.

[21] Wax, M.B., Tezel, G. (2002) Neurobiology of glaucomatous optic neuropathy: diverse cellular events in neurodegeneration and neuroprotection. *Mol. Neurobiol*, 26, 45-55.

[22] Hickey, W.F., Hsu, B.L., Kimura, H. (1991) T-lymphocyte entry into the central nervous system. *J. Neurosci. Res*, 28, 254-260.

[23] Raivich, G., Jones, L.L., Kloss, C.U., et al. (1998) Immune surveillance in the injured nervous system: T-lymphocytes invade the axotomized mouse facial motor nucleus and aggregate around sites of neuronal degeneration. *J. Neurosci*, 18, 5804-5816.

[24] Schwartz, M., Kipnis, J. (2001) Protective autoimmunity: regulation and prospects for vaccination after brain and spinal cord injuries. *Trends Mol. Med*, 7, 252.

[25] Wax, M.B., Tezel, G., Saito, I., Gupta, R.S., Harley, J.B., Li, Z., Romano, C. (1998) Anti-Ro/SS-A positivity and heat shock protein antibodies in patients with normal-pressure glaucoma. *Am. J. Ophthalmol*, 125, 145-157.

[26] Wax, M.B., Barrett, D.A., Pestronk, A. (1994) Increased incidence of paraproteinemia and autoantibodies in patients with normal-pressure glaucoma. *Am. J. Ophthalmol*, 117, 561-568.

[27] Tezel, G., Seigel, G.M., Wax, M.B. (1998) Autoantibodies to small heat shock proteins in glaucoma. *Invest Ophthalmol. Vis. Sci*, 39, 2277-2287.

[28] Tezel, G., Hernandez, R., Wax, M.B. (2000) Immunostaining of heat shock proteins in the retina and optic nerve head of normal and glaucomatous eyes. *Arch Ophthalmol*, 118, 511-518.

[29] Nobrega, A., Haury, M., Grandien, A., Malanchère, E., Sundblad, A., Coutinho, A. (1993) Global analysis of antibody repertoires. II. Evidence for specificity, self-selection and the immunological "homunculus" of antibodies in normal serum. *Eur. J. Immunol*, 23, 2851-2859.

[30] Avrameas, S. (1991) Natural autoantibodies: from 'horror autotoxicus' to 'gnothi seauton'. *Immunol. Today*, 1991, 154-159.

[31] Poletaev, A., Osipenko, L. (2003) General network of natural autoantibodies as immunological homunculus (Immunculus). *Autoimmun. Rev*, 2, 264-271.

[32] Ferreyra, H.A., Jayasundera, T., Khan, N.W., He, S., Lu, Y., Heckenlively, J.R. (2009) Management of autoimmune retinopathies with immunosuppression. *Arch Ophthalmol*, 127, 390-397.

[33] Erlanger, B.F. (1989) Some thoughts on the structural basis of internal imagery. *Immunol. Today*, 10, 151-152.

[34] Zimmermann, C.W., Eblen, F. (1993) Repertoires of autoantibodies against homologous eye muscle in ocular and generalized myasthenia gravis differ. *Clin. Invest*, 71, 445-451.

[35] Zimmermann, C.W., Weiss, G. (1987) Antibodies not directed against the acetylcholine receptor in myasthenia gravis. An immunoblot study. *J. Neuroimmunol*, 16, 225-236.

[36] Grus, F.H., Joachim, S.C., Wuenschig, D., Rieck, J., Pfeiffer, N. (2008) Autoimmunity and glaucoma. *J. Glaucoma*, 17, 79-84.

[37] Morohoshi, K., Goodwin, A.M., Ohbayashi, Y., Ono, S.J. (2009) Autoimmunity in retinal degeneration: autoimmune retinopathy and age-related macular degeneration. *J. Autoimmun.*, 33, 247-254.

[38] Klein, R., Wang, Q., Klein, B.E.K., Moss, S.E., Meuer, S.E. (1995) The relationship of age-related maculopathy, cataract, and glaucoma to visual acuity. *Invest Ophthalmol. Vis. Sci*, 36, 182-191.

[39] Kijlstra, A., La Heij, E., Hendrikse, F. (2005) Immunological factors in the pathogenesis and treatment of age-related macular degeneration. *Ocul. Immunol. Inflamm*, 13, 3-11.

[40] Penfold, P.A., Killingsworth, M.C., Sarks, S.H. (1985) Senile macular degeneration: the involvement of immunocompetent cells. *Graefes Arch Clin. Exp. Ophthalmol*, 223, 69-76.

[41] Anderson, D.H., Mullins, R.F., Hageman, G.S., Johnson, L.V. (2002) A role for local inflammation in the formation of drusen in the aging eye. *Am. J. Ophthalmol*, 134, 411-431.

[42] Mullins R.F., Russell S.R., Anderson, D.H., Hageman, G.S. (2000) Drusen associated with aging and age-related macular degeneration contain proteins common to extracellular deposits associated with atherosclerosis, elastosis, amyloidosis, and dense deposit disease. *FASEB J*, 14, 835-846.

[43] Penfold, P.L., Provis, J.M., Furby, J.H., Gatenby, P.A., Billson, F.A. (1990) Autoantibodies to retinal astrocytes associated with age-related macular degeneration. *Graefe's Arch Clin. Exp. Ophthalmol*, 228, 270-274.

[44] Gurne, D.H., Tso, M.O.M., Edward, D.P., Ripps, H. (1991) Antiretinal antibodies in serum of patients with age-related macular degeneration. *Ophthalmology*, 98, 602–607.

[45] Wang J.J., Mitchell, P., Smith, W., Gillies, M, Billson, F; Blue Mountains Eye Study. (2003) Systemic use of anti-inflammatory medications and age-related maculopathy: the Blue Mountains Eye Study. *Ophthalmic. Epidemiol*, 10, 37-48.

[46] Bielory, L. (2000) Allergic and immunologic disorders of the eye. Part I: Immunology of the eye. *J. Allergy Clin. Immunol.*, 106, 805-816.

[47] Nussenblatt, R.B., Ferris, F. (2007) Age-related macular degeneration and the immune response: implications for therapy. *Am. J. Ophthalmol.*, 144, 618-626.

[48] Chen, J., Connor, K.M., Smith, L.E.H. (2007) Overstaying their welcome: defective $CX_3CR_1$ microglia eyed in macular degeneration. *J. Clin. Invest.*, 117, 2758-2762.

[49] Bora P.S., Hu, Z.W., Tezel, T.H., Sohn, J.H., Kang, S.G., Cruz, J.M.C., Bora, N.S., Garen, A., Kaplan, H.J. (2003) Immunotherapy for choroidal neovascularization in a laser-induced mouse model simulating exudative (wet) macular degeneration. *Proc. Natl. Acad. Sci. USA*, 100, 2679.

In: Immunology in Clinic Practice
Editor: Cagatay Oktenli, pp. 85-114
ISBN 978-1-60876-644-4


*Chapter 6*

# PSYCHONEUROIMMUNOLOGY: LATEST ADVANCES

***Semai Bek[1], Levent Sütcigil[2] and Ali Bozkurt[2]***
1. Department of Neurology,
Gülhane Military Medical Academy, Ankara, Turkey
2. Department of Psychiatry,
Gülhane Military Medical Academy, Ankara, Turkey

## ABSTRACT

Psychoneuroimmunology (PNI) is the study of the interaction between the nervous and immune systems of the human body. The two major units of the body are the central nervous system (CNS) and the immune system. The immune system has often been looked upon as autonomous; however, latest researches provided that the existence of reciprocal communication pathways between the nervous, endocrine, and immune systems. In light of this evidence, there has been a growing interest in the supposed involvement of the immune system in both neurological and psychiatric disorders.

**Keywords:** Psychoneuroimmunology; central nervous system; blood brain barrier; blood-cerebrospinal fluid; chronic stress

## INTRODUCTION

Despite the exceedingly complex biological and structural make up of the CNS, it has a limited repertoire for its own protection but it has the capacity to engage the peripheral immune system to eliminate infection and toxic/metabolic processes [1]. Central nervous system has several protective mechanisms; a) the blood brain barrier (BBB), b) its own immunoregulatory cells like microglia, astrocytes, oligodendrocytes and endothelial cells, c) lack of a lymphatic drainage system [1]. Glial cells present antigen and express major histocompatibility complex (MHC) class I and II [1]. They also regulate production and uptake of excitotoxins, and secrete trophic factors that nurture nervous system cells and protect their critical functions [1].

## Intracerebral Regulation of Immune Responses

For many years, it was thought that the CNS has been shown to be an immune-privileged site due to the lack of lymphatic drainage and dendritic cells and the presence of blood-brain and blood-cerebrospinal fluid (CSF) barriers [2]. But recent evidence suggest that the CNS itself plays a role in inhibiting the activation of immune cells [2]. This is thought to be accomplished by local production of immunosuppressive cytokines and neuropeptides. It has been proposed that neurotrophins and neurotransmitters have been proposed to play a major role in down-regulating the activation state of CNS intrinsic macrophages, the microglia [3]. Immune privilege in the brain is also thought to be actively maintained through immune deviation mechanisms that involve preferential induction of humoral responses to CNS-derived antigens and supression of CNS antigen-specific delayed-type hypersensitivity [4].

## Complement in Central Nervous System

Classically, the complement system provides an innate immune mechanism against pathogens and it can be activated through classical, alternative and lectin pathways [5-10]. All three share the common step of activating the central component C3 [9]. CNS contains proteins of the complement system that are synthesized by astrocytes, microglia, and neurons [5,9]. Microglia can switch from a resting state to an active or reactive state. In addition, it has been reported that bioactive peptides produced through complement activation can mediate a variety of pro-inflammatory responses [9]. In post-mortem studies, small levels of complement activation have been found in young subjects and aged controls [9,10]. Activated microglia have been demonstrated *in vivo* in the Alzheimer's disease patients [9,11,12].

## Cytokines in Central Nervous System

Cytokines comprise a group of polypeptides with many properties shared with hormones and growth factors. Some cytokines mediate and regulate innate immunity, other mediate and regulate specific immunity, some have mainly a pro-inflammatory or an antiinflammatory effect, and other cytokines stimulate haematopoiesis. Different cells may produce the same cytokine, but one cytokine may have different effects in different circumstances. Different cytokines may duplicate or antagonize effects depending on the situation. Many of them are involved in the pathogenesis of neurological disorders [13].

The Guillain-Barré syndrome (GBS) is an acute inflammatory disease mainly affecting the myelin of peripheral nerves. The disease is associated with elevated numbers of myelin-reactive T and B-lymphocytes. The myelin loss may follow or be induced by a direct action of tumor necrosis factor (TNF)-α on Schwann cell membranes [14]. High number of interleukin (IL) 10 secreting blood mononuclear cells early in the course of the disease decrease during the recovery phase [15]. IL-18 has been implicated in GBS [16]. The balance between cytokines with pro- and cytokines with anti-inflammatory effects determine the course of the disease and the end result.

The main symptoms of myasthenia gravis (MG) are caused by the effect of autoantibodies directed against the nicotinic acetylcholine receptor (AChR) of the muscle end plates [17]. The autoantibody production depends on the interaction between the antibody-producing B-lymphocytes and the Th lymphocytes. Th1 cells secrete proinflammatory cytokines like IFNγ while Th2 cells secrete B-stimulatory cytokines such as IL-4. MG is a prototype of an autoantibody-mediated autoimmune disease and it has therefore been believed that Th2 cells promote MG. AChR-reactive IL-10 secreting cells are characteristic for human MG. The serum levels of IL-18 are significantly elevated, and the concentrations are highest in patients with generalized disease and tend to decrease with clinical improvement. Antibodies to IFNα and IL-12 seem to be specific for the presence of a thymoma in MG [17]. It is unknown whether cytokines have a direct effect on the neuromuscular transmission.

Rasmussen's encephalitis is the only form of epilepsy where immune mechanisms mechanisms have been shown to be involved in the pathogenesis. There is evidence that Rasmussen's encephalitis has autoimmune markers, probably characterized by an immune response against the glutamate receptor GluR3 [18]. Several cytokines may be involved in reactive gliosis, axonal sprouting, enhanced neurogenesis and neuronal cell death [19].

## Neurotrophic Cross-talk between the Immune and Central Nervous System

Conceptually, the immune and nervous systems need to relay information across very short and very long distances [20]. The nervous system communicates over both long and short ranges primarily by means of more or less hardwired intercellular connections. In the immune system, long-range communication occurs mainly via the ordered and guided migration of immune cells and soluble factors (cytokines, chemokines and antibodies). On the other hand, short-range communication is mediated by locally acting soluble factors and/or transpires during direct cell–cell contact across specialized areas [20]. These parallels in intercellular communication are complemented by a complex array of factors that induce cell growth and differentiation. In this way, these factors in the immune system are called cytokines; in the nervous system, they are called neurotrophic factors [20]. Some of the most potent members of the neurotrophin family like nerve growth factor (NGF) and brain-derived neurotrophic factor (BDNF), act on or are produced by immune cells [20,21]. These factors may allow the two systems to "cross-talk".

## B Cells in Central Nervous System

It is well known that B cells are involved in the pathophysiology of a number of neurological disorders [22] and they are also capable of responding to an antigen within the CNS [23]. B cells constitutively express the adhesion molecules and during an immune demyelinating process, facilitates their transmigration within the CNS [24-28]. The role of B cells and antibodies in demyelination process appear to be involved in different stages of the disease or subgroups of MS [25]. After therapeutic plasmapheresis, the improvement of the patients supports this concept [26]. High B cell numbers are also reported in the CSF of MS patients and correlate with the rate of disease progression [29]. In MS patients, intrathecal production of IgM anti-myelin antibodies also appears to be a predictor of aggressive evolution [30]. In MS lesions, memory B cells and upregulation of co-stimulatory molecules like CD80 have been suggested [31]. Antibodies against myelin oligodendrocyte glycoprotein (MOG), which are specific for myelin proteins, may play a role in the initiation or progression of the inflammatory process in MS [32-35].

Myasthenia gravis (MG) is a prototypic B cell-mediated autoimmune disease caused by pathogenic antibodies directed against the muscle AchR [36]. Anti- MuSk antibodies are found in a subset of patients with AChR negative MG [37]. Lambert-Eaton myasthenic syndrome (LEMS) is characterised by antibodies directed against VGCC at the presynaptic nerve terminals [36]. Neuromyotonia and non-paraneoplastic limbic encephalitis are characterized by antibodies to VGKC [38]. Neuromyotonia and limbic encephalitis respond to plasmapheresis, intravenous immunoglobulin (IVIg) or immunosuppressive agents [39].

Guillain-Barré syndrome is characterised by 4 main subtypes: acute inflammatory demyelinating polyneuropathy (AIDP); acute motor axonal neuropathy (AMAN); acute motor sensory axonal neuropathy (AMSAN); and Miller Fisher syndrome (MFS). The implicated antigens for these subtypes may be different because it has been suggested that the immune attack appears to be directed at different targets: Schwann cell surface membrane or the myelin in AIDP, the axonal membrane in motor fibres in AMAN, both motor and sensory nerve fibres in AMSAN, and nodal regions of the ocular motor nerve and distal nerve terminals in MFS [40-42].

Chronic, antibody-associated demyelinating polyneuropathies have 3 main subsets: multifocal motor neuropathy (MMN), CIDP and IgM anti-myelin-associated glycoprotein (MAG) demyelinating neuropathy [43]. In CIDP, the implicated antibodies are directed against glycolipids, GM1 or Po [44]. In anti-MAG neuropathies, the antibodies are directed against MAG or glycolipids [44,45].

## Macrophages in Central Nervous System

Classically, macrophages eliminate pathogens or unwanted cells from the body [46]. Pro-inflammatory cytokines, free radicals, glutamate and metalloproteases, which are products of activated macrophages, have some effects on neurodegeneration [46]. It has been reported that TNF-α increases axonal vulnerability by enhancing demyelination via oligodendrocyte killing [47]. *In vitro*, a role for cytokines in initiation of glutamate-induced neuronal damage is also suggested for IL-1 and IL-6, but several studies indicate that IL-6 may have a neuroprotective effect [46].

Reactive oxygen species (ROS) are released in high concentrations by the oxidative burst of macrophages during inflammation [46,48]. It has been suggested that markers of oxidative stress were high in patients with MS [49]. NO products are detectable in serum and CSF of MS patients [50]. Glutamate levels were reported to be increased [51] and the expression of glutamate receptors was reported to be altered in MS in the CSF of MS patients [52]. MMPs are produced by inflammatory cells to degrade the extracellular matrix to facilitate their migration into the CNS [46]. It has been reported that MMPs are found in acute lesions of MS [46]. In addition, a direct role for MMP-9 in neuronal dysfunction has been suggested [53].

## Chemokines in Central Nervous System

In addition to their well-known role in the function of the immune system, chemokines also exert important functions in the CNS [54]. Numerous *in vitro* studies have suggested that chemokines are expressed in the CNS by astrocytes, microglial cells, and neurons [54]. Chemokines play a crucial role in the modulation of synaptic activity in the brain. These proteins regulate the leukocyte infiltration in the brain during neuroinflammatory conditions and diseases [54].A recent study examined the expression levels of chemokines and chemokine receptors on cells in the CSF as well as in brain tissues obtained from MS patients [55]. It has been reported that the IL-8, produced in reperfusion following transient ischemia, contributes to tissue damage, whereas an anti-IL-8 neutralizing antibody significantly reduced brain edema and infarct size [56]. The presence of the CXCR3 chemokine receptor has been reported in neurons and neuronal processes in various cortical and subcortical regions in Alzheimer's disease (AD) brain [57]. MCP-1 is potent microglial and macrophage chemoattractants *in vitro* [58].

## Immunology in Cholinergic Anti-inflammatory Pathway

Accumulating evidence suggest that vagus nerve signaling inhibits cytokine activities and improves disease endpoints in experimental models of sepsis, ischemia/reperfusion, hemorrhagic shock, experimental arthritis, ileus, pancreatitis, and myocardial ischemia [59-67]. Acetylcholine (ACh), the major vagus nerve neurotransmitter, may play a role in the cellular molecular mechanism for inhibition of cytokine synthesis [68,69]. Macrophages and other cytokine-producing cells express AChRs [68,69]. The vagus nerve–derived cholinergic signals provide tonic or continuous neurological modulation of cytokine synthesis [69]. Depressed vagus nerve activity might facilitate the inflammatory responses underlying and worsening disease [70].

## Immunology in Multiple Sclerosis

In MS there must be an alteration in an individual's immune system, resulting in a loss of immunologic tolerance to myelin components. There are several mechanisms for loss of tolerance to self antigens. There can be a change in regulatory cells that normally control responses to autologous proteins. This change must be specific for antimyelin regulatory cells since there is no general dysregulation of immune responses in persons with MS. Loss of regulatory cells, in the form of suppressor cells, was first described in 1978. The concept of a pure suppressor cell is not demonstrated and the concept of a pathologically relevant loss of regulatory cells in MS has not yet been sustained [71].

Another possibility is that in MS immunocompetent cells appear that are able to recognize myelin antigens. In MS, the patterns of response to myelin antigens are less well defined. There may be different forms of myelin destruction in different individuals that is that MS is not one disease but a syndrome, with myelin destruction as the final common pathway [72]. If this is the case, there is the theoretical possibility that administration of agents resulting in a Th1 to Th2 shift could be ineffective and unresponsiveness to treatment is all too often seen in persons with MS.

Third is the possibility that immune responses to myelin antigens that are normally immunologically sequestered are exposed to an MS patient's immune system, resulting in additional damage to myelin with release of additional myelin antigens, leading to the phenomenon of epitope spreading, a cascading of immune responses to the additional antigens. Most frequently mentioned is MBP. Other myelin antigens also are implicated in the pathogenesis of MS. These include MOG, proteolipid protein (PLP), and cyclic nucleotide phosphodiesterase (CNP) [73]. The issue of finding the inciting antigen in MS is complicated by the phenomenon of epitope spreading in which an immune response to an initiating antigen diversifies or spreads to involve responses to adjacent antigens as tissues are destroyed and new antigens are released.

These data support a prominent role for immune mechanisms in MS-related tissue destruction and also that there may be a continuum between the changes induced by an antibrain CNS immune response and processes of tissue destruction not directly related to systemic immune system activity. The existing data do not definitively establish that MS is an autoimmune disease. The strongest datum supporting at least a partial role for immune-mediated tissue destruction in MS is the fact that all currently proven treatments for MS are believed to exert their beneficial effects by modulating immune system function [74].

The rationale for the use of immunosuppressants in MS relies on the hypothesis, supported by a large amount of preclinical and clinical observations, that MS is primarily an inflammatory cell-mediated autoimmune disease. A crucial concept is that inflammation is not only a detrimental event in the pathophysiology of MS, but that it can also act to protect the CNS and enhance repair. The overall interest in the use of immunosuppressant drugs is growing. On the basis of previous unexpected results with other MS treatments which failed despite encouraging pre-clinical evidence and a strong rationale, caution should always be exercised concerning a particular combination therapy until definite evidence of its effectiveness has been achieved [75].

Mitoxantrone is an anthracenedione and initially used as an antineoplastic drug since it interacts with topoisomerase-2 and acts as a DNA intercalating agent. Mitoxantrone has a potent immunosuppressive effect, acting both on B and T cells and reducing levels of several pro-inflammatory cytokines [76]. The use of mitoxantrone in the treatment of MS was approved by the FDA, and confirmed also by a Cochrane review [77]. The cardiotoxicity of mitoxantrone is probably due to the intracellular generation of reactive oxygen intermediated via iron or enzyme-mediated oxidation-reduction reactions in myocardiocytes. Molecule modification recently led to the discovery of pixantrone, a less-cardiotoxic mitoxantrone analogue [78]. A second major and worrying side effect is acute leukemia.

Azathioprine antagonizes purine metabolism and may inhibit the synthesis of DNA, RNA, and proteins; it may also interfere with cellular metabolism and inhibit mitosis. The results of the most recent revision of available meta-analyses of azathioprine use in MS evidenced that the annual relapse rate after one, two or three years was significantly better in the treated patients [79]. The most frequently reported side effects were leukopenia, anorexia, diarrhea and vomiting, abdominal pain with gastrointestinal disturbances, abnormal liver function and skin rashes.

Cyclophosphamide's cytotoxic action is primarily due to a cross-linking of strands of DNA and RNA, as well as to the inhibition of protein synthesis. Given the potential severity of cyclophosphamide early side effects (mainly alopecia, gastrointestinal intolerance and leukopenia with sepsis), and particularly of the long term risk of urinary bladder cancer, its use has been limited in recent years to aggressive or refractory MS forms, frequently in combination with other agents. On the basis of the available results, cyclophosphamide is a therapeutic option as a rescue therapy for patients who are non-responders to IFNb or GA, although its effectiveness as a single agent has not yet been clearly established [80].

The results of the reported trials do not support a noteable clinical effect of methotrexate, although some benefit in performance scores and in MRI results has been reported [81]. The combination of methotreaxate and IFNb-1a is investigated with some positive effects in an open-label trial [82]. The major safety concern in the use of methotrexate is liver toxicity.

Corticosteroids are commonly used in the treatment of MS relapses to shorten their duration and to reduce their severity, although the type of drug, optimal dose, frequency, duration of treatment and route of administration are stil debated. The combination of methylprednisolone and IFNb is safe and well tolerated. Chronic corticosteroid administration is associated with a risk of diabetes, hypertension, osteoporosis, liver function impairment, psychosis, infections and cataract, while pre-existing diseases may be worsened. Anaphylactoid reactions may also occur occasionally [75].

Cladribine is an adenosine deaminase-resistant purine nucleoside causing an accumulation of deoxynucleotides in lymphocytes. Despite the fact that no toxic side effects have been reported, the long term safety of cladribine, a drug which acts by being incorporated into DNA, may still is a cause for concern.

Mycophenolate mofetil is a selective inhibitor of inosine 5'-monophosphate dehydrogenase type II, and through this mechanism it is able to reduce their activity during inflammation. In the treatment of MS, mycophenolate mofetil has been used primarily in SPMS, but also in refractory RRMS and PPMS patients. It is well tolerated, although gastrointestinal side effects and alteration in liver enzymes have been reported. The results in terms of efficacy are less clear [83].

Intravenous immunoglobulins may also be effective in the treatment of MS [84]. Adverse effects during IVIg treatment were very rare and mild: in most cases they comprised transient skin reactions, headache and fever. A different use of IVIgs regards the possibility of preventing an increase in MS relapse rate immediately after pregnancy [85]. However, further randomized double-blind studies are needed to confirm their effectiveness.

It has been demonstrated that patients with severe attacks of MS may improve rapidly after plasma exchange treatment. Plasma exchange seems effective in a subgroup of patients with severe relapses resistance to methylprednisolone therapy [86]. Another possible indication for the use of plasma exchange was suggested by a recent report of its efficacy in severe optic neuritis [87].

Autologous bone marrow transplantation (BMT) and autologous hematopoietic stem cell transplantation (HSCT) may be an option for the most severe cases of MS which are resistant to any other less aggressive treatment [88,89]. The procedure is feasible in MS and that it decreases the clinical severity of the disease, a result supported also by the MRI results. The high incidence of severe side effects and the high mortality rate still remain the main limitations to a wider use of HSCT and are a major challenge in the design and evaluation of future trials [90]. Several new immunosuppressant drugs, intracellular ligands, cell surface ligands and anti-cytokines are under investigation [75,91].

## Autoimmune and Paraneoplastic Channelopathies

Autoimmune channelopathies are a group of paraneoplastic neurological disorders associated with antibodies to specific ion channels on neurons or muscle [92]. Autoimmune autonomic ganglionopathy (AAG), appears to be due to antibody-mediated disruption of synaptic transmission in autonomic ganglia. Patients with AAG have high titers of autoantibodies directed against the ganglionic (alpha3-type) AChR [93]. Testing for ganglionic AChR antibodies has allowed the identification of additional cases with insidious symptom onset. Such chronic cases may be initially indistinguishable from degenerative forms of autonomic failure but can respond to treatment [94,95]. Episodic ataxia type 1 (EA1) is a rare autosomal dominant disorder caused by mutation in the Kv1.1 channel [96]. Autoimmune neuromyotonia (Isaacs' syndrome) is an acquired disorder. Encephalopathy, seizures, sleep disturbances, or behavioral changes may represent the effects of VGKC antibodies on neuronal excitability in the CNS [97,98]. Antibodies against Kv1.6 and Kv1.2 appear to be most relevant in neuromyotonia and limbic encephalitis [99].

Unique features of limbic encephalitis with VGKC antibodies are the frequent association with hyponatremia [39,100]. The rapid response to plasma exchange suggests a direct role of the antibodies [39].

Rasmussen encephalitis is a severe form of intractable childhood epilepsy and encephalopathy. Antibodies against one subtype of neuronal AMPA-type glutamate receptor (GluR3) and neuronal alpha7-type AChR are thought to be responsible [101].

It has been reported that many patients with neuromyelitis optica have antibodies against aquaporin-4, a membrane water channel found in the CNS [34]. Aquaporin antibodies help to identify patients with NMO and direct treatment. NMO may represent a novel form of autoimmune channelopathy [102].

## Tumor Immunology and Target Immunotherapy for Central Nervous System Malignancies

Immunotherapeutic manipulations that have yielded promising results for peripherally located tumors do not, in turn, result in similar efficacy for the same tumors located within the confines of the CNS [103,104]. Thus, new treatment strategies must find ways to augment existing immunotherapeutics. Immune-based treatments for disease generally fall into two categories: passive immunotherapy or active immunotherapy [103].

In passive immunotherapy, immunity is exogenously "transferred" by injection of either T cells or antibodies specific for an antigen. Thus, an individual passively acquires immunity, thereby not having to effectively generate immunity using endogenous immune cells. It is suitable if the patient is severely immunocompromised. Serotherapy is a form of passive immunotherapy that involves the administration of antigen-specific antibodies. Tumor-specific antibodies used to target CNS glioma cells and deliver radiochemicals or immunotoxins to the tumor site have been investigated extensively [105,106]. Experiences with radiolabeled anti-tenascin monoclonal antibody (mAb) 81C6 have resulted in increases in survival and prolonged disease stabilization [106]. Clinical trials of immunotoxins for CNS neoplasia have been conducted with 454A12-RA (an anti-transferrin mAb plus recombinant ricin A chain immunotoxin), TFN-CRM107 (human diferric transferrin plus Diphtheria toxin mutant CRM107), and IL-4-PE38KDEL (IL-4 plus Pseudomonas aeruginosa exotoxin A mutant PE38KDEL) [103]. These initial trials of passive serotherapy have shown some significant antitumor effects, which have spurred further multicenter Phase II/III trials using radiolabeled or immunotoxin-conjugated antibodies as therapeutic approaches for human brain tumors. Adoptive transfer of lymphokine-activated killer (LAK) cells, tumor-infiltrating lymphocytes, and expanded systemic T cells have also been used to treat patients with malignant glioma but no consistent results were available [103].

Active (vaccine) immunotherapy seeks to generate or augment endogenous host immunity by specifically boosting the host's own immune response to an antigen. Tumor cells have been transduced to express various immune-enhancing cytokines, MHC antigens, or costimulatory molecules and used to vaccinate tumor-bearing animals and patients [103]. This "immuno-gene therapy" strategy attempts to augment the immune response with genetic modification. Cytokine-based tumor cell vaccination has been investigated for brain tumors [107]. This approach often involves the introduction of cytokine genes (such as interferons and interleukins) into neoplastic cells. Another active immunotherapeutic approach involves the use of DC, which can also augment the host immune response to foreign antigens.

Phase I/II clinical trials are currently under way [103]. Although the information offered by clinical data to date are too limited to draw any conclusions about.

## Immunotherapy for Paraneoplastic Neurological Disorders

In paraneoplastic encephalomyelitis, tumor treatment offers the best chance of stabilizing the patient's neurological condition, while immunotherapy does not appear to modify the outcome of the disease [108]. Plasma exchange, IVIG, and corticosteroids have limited efficacy, therefore, more aggressive immunosuppression with cyclophosphamide, tacrolimus, or cyclosporine may be considered [109,-111].

Paraneoplastic limbic encephalitis (PLE) is a rare disorder characterized by the subacute onset of short-term memory loss, confusion, and seizures suggesting involvement of the limbic system [112]. It has been reported that immunotherapy is largely ineffective.

Paraneoplastic cerebellar degeneration is one of the most common and characteristic PNS and incidental improvement has been reported in association with plasma exchange, rituximab, steroids or IVIg [113].

Opsoclonus is a disorder of ocular motility that consists of arrhythmic, involuntary, high-amplitude conjugate saccades in all directions [114]. Improvement following the administration of plasma exchange, plasma filtration with a protein A column, steroids, cyclophosphamide, azathioprine or IVIG has been reported [114].

## Intravenous Immunoglobulin in Neurological Disorders

MS is the most common autoimmune disease of the CNS. Although high-dose glucocorticosteroid regimen does not improve symptoms in many cases, IVIG application during a relapse as concomitant therapy to methylprednisolone does not further shorten relapse duration [115]. However, IVIG prolong the time to the second relapse in MS patients with a first attack [116]. In relapsing–remitting MS, long-term IVIG application is able to reduce the relapse rate, and also has beneficial effects on disease progression [84]. The investigation of IVIG in chronic progressive MS did not yield positive results [117].

In adult GBS, controlled studies proved the efficacy of high-dose IVIG, but the combination with glucocorticosteroids does not improve overall outcomes [118]. On the other hand, in the Miller–Fisher variant of GBS, IVIG is not superior to supportive therapy alone [119]. In patients with CIDP, IVIG led to a persistent therapeutic effect [120]. IVIG may also be beneficial in cases of treatment-resistant vasculitic peripheral neuropathy and diabetic neuropathy [121,122]. In MMN, controlled trials were investigated the effect of IVIG [123].

In MG, researches suggested that the length of stay in the hospital was shorter and a significant improvement was observed in muscle strength in the IVIG group [124,125]. However, in chronic MG, little evidence are available for the application of IVIG.

The application of IVIG in polymyositis is not well studied. Inclusion body myositis is characterized by degenerative changes in association with strong inflammation. One study disclosed stabilization or even mild improvement of patients under IVIG therapy [126].

## Plasma Exchange in Neuroimmunological Disorders

Therapeutic plasma exchange (TPE) removes antibodies and substances leading to immune mediated disorders. In immune mediated neurological disorders, TPE is often used alone or in combination with other treatment options [127-132]. TPE therapy has some potential complications [128]. The Cochrane Systematic meta-analysis reported that TPE was the only treatment for GBS found to be superior to supportive treatment [133].

In MG, some non-randomized studies reported that TPE is beneficial in the short-term outcome of disease. There is no adequate randomized, controlled trial to determine whether TPE improves neither short-term nor long-term outcome for MG [134].

There are some case reports in which TPE could be effective after corticosteroid failure in demyelinating disorders [135,136].

# Psychiatric Perspectives of Brain, Behavior, and the Immune System

The increasing insight regarding the interaction between the immune system and the neuroendocrine system gained in the last few decades has shown that this interaction plays a role in many diseases such as sepsis, rheumatologic diseases, autoimmune diseases, cardiac diseases, neurological diseases, and psychiatric disorders [137-139].

The immune system is regulated by the central nervous system (CNS) through neuronal and neuroendocrine pathways. Consecutively, the immune system signals the brain via neural and humoral routes. Immune organs are innervated by the sympathetic nervous system and immune cells express receptors for neurotransmitters including catecholamines, neuropeptides, and for hormones [140,141]. Additionally, via the vagus nerve, the parasympathetic system contributes to the bidirectional connection between the brain and the immune system [142].

## Immune System

The mammalian immune system not only protects the organism from a diverse collection of pathogenic mechanisms but also avoids giving responses that produce excessive damage of self-tissues. Since our environment comprises a wide range of pathogenic organisms with a broad selection of pathologic mechanisms, the immune response utilizes a complex protective mechanism so as to control and eradicate these pathogens. The mechanism aims to detect the structural features of the pathogens and to mark them as being separate from host cells [143].

Mechanisms either recognize the molecular patterns by hard-wired responses that are encoded by genes in the host's germ line or by means of responses that are encoded by gene elements that somatically rearrange to result in the assembly of antigen-binding molecules [143]. The former comprises the innate immune response and is able to respond to microbial infections rapidly. It acts as a first response against invading pathogens after the development of the adaptive immune response. The latter comprises the adaptive immune response which develops in reaction to an infection by the selection of B- and T-lymphocytes. Due to the vast number of potential antigens, the adaptive immune system generates very few cells with specificity for each antigen [143].

After they are activated, the responding cells need to proliferate so as to provide an adequate response. This is why this response is much more specific than the innate immune system. However, it is also much slower. After repeated exposures to the antigen, it is able to react faster and more vigorously due to its ability to memorize the response to a specific antigen [144]. Although the innate and adaptive immune systems differ to a great extent in terms of the rapidity and specificity of the response, there is crosstalk between both mechanisms [143].

## Regulation of Immunity

As changes in immune system structure and function are associated with both stress and behavioral conditioning, it is proposed that the cells of the immune system are influenced by mediators released from the nervous and/or endocrine systems. A number of recent articles have documented and discussed the evidence in support of the existence of a neuroimmune connection [145-148].

The hypothalamic-pituitary-adrenal axis comprises the neuroendocrine system that controls reactions to stress and has important functions in regulating various body processes [149].

Both human and animal primary and secondary lymphoid organs are innervated with sympathetic nerve fibers [150,151]. While acetylcholine potently modulates several classical immune reactions via the vagus nerve, the sympathetic nervous system can alter the Th1/Th2 balance through stimulation of the beta adrenergic receptor [152].

Adrenergic receptors bind catecholamines like norepinephrine and epinephrine [153]. Initially, radioligand binding analyses that were performed on isolated subsets of innate immune cells showed that all cells expressed the $\beta_2$AR [152]. These findings were recently confirmed by analyses of mRNA expression [154]. However, whether other βAR subtypes are expressed by PMN remains unclear.

## Cytokines

The autonomic nervous system (ANS) is capable of modulating peripheral cytokine production. The ANS may influence immunocompetent cells through parasympathetic innervation of the immune system organs. Sympathetic nerve fibres signal the immune system via NA release from the peripheral sympathetic ganglia. The parasympathetic vagal nucleus may down regulate cytokine production through ACh signaling by the vagus nerve [142]. On the other hand, exposure to psychological stress has also been accounted for influencing proinflammatory cytokine production [155]. In this sense, HPA axis activity are also involved [156].

In addition to infiltration or indirect signaling from the periphery, cytokines have been reported to be constitutively produced in the CNS itself, mainly by astrocytes and microglia [157]. Under certain conditions, neurons are also assumed to be able to release cytokines. Cytokine production has been found to occur in several brain sites such as basal ganglia, forebrain regions, circumventricular regions, hypothalamus, hippocampus, cerebellum and brainstem nuclei [158].

## Behavioral Effects of Cytokines

Peripheral and central administration of IL-1α, IL-1β, and TNF-α to healthy laboratory animals induces activation of the HPA axis and behavioral symptoms of sickness. With regards to the central amine variations induced by the cytokines, it is proposed that immune activation may influence complex behavioral processes and affective state [159].

Cytokines have been shown to affect many behaviors such as sleep, appetite, sexual behavioral, memory, and motor activity. Cytokines are accountable for behaviors displayed during infectious disease, referred to as sickness behavior. The symptoms in sickness behavior such as lethargy, somnolence, fatigue, lack of interest, lack of appetite, decreased concentration, is similar to many symptoms described in the depressive syndrome [160]. Depressed activity and apathy are commonly observed along with reduction in food intake. Social exploration and food intake are the two behavioral patterns that have been mostly used to explore what the mechanisms of cytokine-induced sickness behavior are.

## Depressed Mood Caused by Immune Activation

In studies regarding the depressive effects of cytokines, it was revealed that, even though all patients responded to the treatment by showing behavioral symptoms of sickness, an important number of them also developed mood disorders [161, 162]. These observations were carried out in patients given cytokine immunotherapy (e.g., IFN-α, IL-2) for the treatment of cancer and viral infections. Cancer patients display relatively pure depressive disorders whereas hepatitis C patients develop episodes of depression alternating with episodes of manic symptoms [163]. In all cases, these psychiatric symptoms develop over a background of neurovegetative sickness symptoms including fatigue, decreased appetite, and sleep disorders. The importance of individual vulnerability factors was shown by the fact that mood disorders occur only in about one-third of the patients receiving immunotherapy. Patients who have clinically diagnosed depressed mood at baseline, before the initiation of immunotherapy, are more at risk than patients with normal mood scores [164]. It is yet unknown if these features are displayed by patients who have the usual risk factors for mood disorders or for a differential activation of the innate immune response.

Proinflammatory cytokines and serotonergic homeostasis have been linked with the pathophysiology of major psychiatric disorders. It has been suggested that Th1, Th2 and Th3 cytokine profile are altered in depressed patients and some of them corrected by sertraline therapy [165].

## Immunological Research in Psychiatry

Psychoneuroimmunology investigates the interactions between behavior and the immune system. The concept of neuroimmune communication includes the immune and the nervous system distinguishes new neuroimmunoloy from its predecessor.

Felten et al. proved that lymphoid organs were innervated by the sympathetic nerve fibers [166]. Moreover, they suggested that nerve terminals were closely associated with lymphocytes. It was proposed that lymphocytes can directly receive neural inputs from the autonomics nervous system.

Empirical studies implicated the pineal gland as a tissue bridging the immune, central nervous and endocrine systems [167]. The pineal gland secretes melatonin, a substance which affects antibody response. This indicated that the pineal gland was functioning as an endocrine tissue.

Cytokines were the focus of the studies carried out in the last two decades. The CNS and immune cells are two systems which can be linked in terms of their ability to secrete and to respond to cytokines. At the same period, the first evidence was discovered. How molecules the size of cytokines could cross the BBB could be explained by the presence of transporters.

Sickness behavior is caused by proinflammatory cytokines that are released during the response to neoplastically transformed cells and/or the damage they engender. Depressed mood, fatigue anhedonia, anorexia, psychomotor slowing, sleep disturbances social isolation, cognitive dysfunction, and increased sensitivity to pain (hyperalgesia) are among its behavioral symptoms [169].

Relevant to understanding the pathophysiology and ultimate treatment of sickness behavior, an explosion of interest has focused on exploring how proinflammatory cytokines insitgate changes in the brain and in behavior [169].

Since the 2000s, evidence has supported that the afferent vagal pathway accumulated significantly. Studies have indicated that peritoneal injection of IL-1 or LPS induced fever was blocked by vagotomy [170]. Other studies suggest that neuroimmune communication is not mediated by a single dominant pathway [171]. The medullary visceral zone was identified as a neural station relating vagal signals to the paraventricular nucleus of hypothalamus [172].

Stimulation of vagal efferents strongly inhibited the production of TNF and protected animals from LPS induced endotoxic shock [173]. They found that the nicotinic acetylcholine α 7 receptor mediates these anti-inflammatory effects [174]. Consequently, immune activities throughout the soma can be sensed by the nervous system and the function of the immune system can be regulated via both sympathetic and parasympathetic outflows. Additionally, acetylcholine α-7 receptor has been discovered in sympathetic postganglionic neurons. As a result, it is possible that it is not the parasympathetic but the sympathetic outflow that wields anti-inflammatory effects.

Findings in the last two decades have noticeably illustrated that neuroimmune communication exists via multiple pathways, and that both neural and humoral pathways play an active role in relating information between the nervous and immune systems [175].

## Brain-Immune Interactions and Implications in Psychiatric Disorders

Research on brain-immune interactions has shed light on the bidirectional connections between the neural and neuroendocrine systems and the immune system. The central nervous system regulates the immune system through neuronal and neuroendocrine pathways and the immune system signals the brain through neural and humoral routes.

The immune system can also signal the CNS through the action of cytokines [176]. These cytokines are produced in the periphery by a variety of immune cells such as monocytes, macrophages, activated T cells, B cells, natural killer (NK) cells, and fibroblast. In addition, cytokines are also produced in the CNS by micraglia, astrocytes, vascular endothelial cells, and fibroblasts [177].

Cytokines can bind to receptors on paraganglia cells near the vagus nerve. They activate the vagus nerve and the brainstem region where the vagus projects, the nucleus tractus solitarius. Cytokines can also exert effects on CRH-producing neurons in the median eminence which activates hypothalamic neurons [177].

Complex components of the immune response including the innate and adaptive immune responses are coordinated in the periphery by cytokines. Cytokines are responsible for neuroendocrine and neuronal activation in the brain. They regulate glial cell growth and proliferation, modulate activity of endogenous opioid peptides, and activate the HPA axis [178]. Additionally, cytokines can affect noradrenergic, serotoninergic, and dopaminergic system metabolism.

Sound evidence points out to the role of cytokines in depression. Cytokines have been shown to affect many behaviors including sleep, appetite, sexual behavioral, memory, and motor activity. Cytokines are accountable for behaviors shown during infectious disease, referred to collectively as sickness behavior. Interestingly, the constellation of symptoms in sickness behavior, such as lethargy, somnolence, fatigue, lack of interest, lack of appetite, decreased concentration, is similar to many symptoms described in the depressive syndrome [160].

The fact that administration of interferon alfa in humans for treatment of infectious disease or cancer can lead to mood disorders including depressive syndromes, manic states, hypomania, and mixed states supports the role of cytokines in depression [163]. In cytokine related depression, symptoms resolve after the cessation of the treatment, or with the use of antidepressants. Prophylactic treatments with antidepressants have prevented depressive episodes in patients receiving cytokines for cancer and other diseases [163]. Moreover, increased risk for depression and reduced responsiveness to antidepressant therapy has been associated with polymorphism of IL-1β and TNF-α genes [179]. Results have also been reported showing no correlation between polymorphism of IL-10, IL-6 and TNF-β genes and depression [180].

Research has shown that levels of proinflammatory cytokines are increased in patients with depression [181]. However, contradictory results have also been described [182]. When potential moderating factors such as age, gender, body mass index, smoking habits, prior medication, and psychiatric comorbidities have been included in the analysis, the association between cytokine levels and MDD is attenuated [183].

Further studies have shown that, after clinical remission in patients with depression, cytokines remain elevated [181] although conflicting results have also been described [184].

Important implications like maintenance of increased pro-inflammatory cytokine levels increase the risk of developing osteoporosis, diabetes, and atherosclerosis [185].

Some investigators have blamed antidepressants for the inhibition of the production of pro-inflammatory cytokines and the stimulation of the production of anti-inflammatory cytokines [186]. On the other hand, in patients with depression, controversial results on the change of cytokine patterns before and after treatment have also been reported [187].

Although conflicting results have also been described [188], positive correlations between some pro-inflammatory cytokines and the presence and intensity of depressive and anxiety symptoms have been described [181]. The connection between depression and increased pro-inflammatory cytokine cannot be overlooked as well as the role of stress in inducing depression. It is obvious that psychological stress is related to and can trigger depression. In human and animal studies, it has already been shown that psychological stress has been associated with increased pro-inflammatory cytokines [189].

## Effects of Stress on the Immune System

The duration and the course of the stress are key factors in determining the nature of stress-induced immune change. [190]. Short-term stressors augment certain aspects of immune function and this can be either beneficial or detrimental in different conditions. Clearly, the influence of acute stress on the immune system is a complex interaction. However, it is a well known fact that chronic or excessive stress has a deleterious effect on immunity [191-198].

Although it was speculated that changes in the immune system might be a relevant mechanism linking stress and morbidity, one of the most severe psychological stressors, conjugal bereavement, was found to be associated with robust declines in cellular immune responses [193].

Psychological stress such as anxiety and depression and the accompanying negative emotions can negatively affect B- and T-cell- mediated immune responses. Psychological stress can also impair the immune response to several antiviral/bacterial vaccines [195, 199, 201].

In persons with easy life style and mental health condition, high levels of blood NK and lymphocyte-activated killer activity were reported. Physical activity would enhance the quantity and quality of blood CD $16^{+}$ NK, and, consecutively, improve mental health by controlling anxiety and depression. These have been linked to depressive disorders in young adults [202]. Persons who were psychologically less capable of coping with such stressful circumstances showed greater decrease in the activity of their NK cells, and lymphocyte proliferation to mitogens [203].

Several studies have also illustrated that individuals' susceptibility to respiratory tract infection, and acceleration of progression to AIDS in HIV-positive men can be altered by stress [195,204]. Stress can provoke increases in proinflammatory cytokines that are associated with a variety of diseases including cardiovascular disease, rheumatoid arthritis, and types 1 and 2 diabetes [205-209].

## CONCLUSION

All recent findings show that peripheral and CNS immune regulatory responses can play ameliatory and harmful roles for disease. Essential to all of this is the challenge for future studies to establish how neural immunity can be harnessed in order to decelerate or abrogate disease by focusing immune responses toward its amelioration and devastation. The increased knowledge of the mechanisms underlying the immune-mediated events leading to neurological diseases has allowed new approaches to the treatment of the disease to be hypothesized. Several new immunosuppressant drugs, intracellular ligands, cell surface ligands and anti-cytokines are under investigation.

## REFERENCES

[1] Gendelman, H.E. (2002) Neural immunity: Friend or foe? *Neurovirol*, 8, 474-479.

[2] Aloisi, F., Ambrosini, E., Columba-Cabezas, S., Magliozzi, R., Serafini, B. (2001) Intracerebral regulation of immune responses. *Ann. Med*, 33, 510-515.

[3] Hoek, R.M., Ruuls, S.R., Murphy, C.A., Wright, G.J., Goddard, R., Zurawski, S.M., Blom, B., Homola, M.E., Streit, W.J., Brown, M.H., Barclay, A.N., Sedgwick, J.D. (2000) Down-regulation of the macrophage lineage through interaction with OX2 (CD200). *Science*, 290, 1768-1771.

[4] Wenkel, H., Streilein, J.W., Young, M.J. (2000) Systemic immune deviation in the brain that does not depend on the integrity of the blood-brain barrier. *J. Immunol*, 164, 5125-5131.

[5] Morley, B.J., Walport, M.J. (2000). The complement system. In: Morley, B.J., Walport, M.J. (Eds.), The Complement Facts Book. Academic Press, London, pp. 7–22.

[6] Arlaud, G.J., Gaboriaud, C., Thielens, N.M., Budayova-Spano M, Rossi V, Fontecilla-Camps JC. (2002) Structural biology of the C1 complex of complement unveils the mechanisms of its activation and proteolytic activity. *Mol. Immunol*, 39, 383–394.

[7] Kishore, U., Gaboriaud, C., Waters, P., Shrive, A.K., Greenhough, T.J., Reid, K.B., Sim, R.B., Arlaud, G.J. (2004) C1q and tumor necrosis factor superfamily: modularity and versatility. *Trends Immunol*, 25, 551–561.

[8] Fujita, T., Matsushita, M., Endo, Y. (2004) The lectin-complement pathway--its role in innate immunity and evolution. *Immunol. Rev*, 198, 185–202.

[9] Bonifati, D.M., Kishore, U. (2007) Role of complement in neurodegeneration and neuroinflammation. *Mol. Immunol*, 44, 999-1010.

[10] Loeffler, D.A., Camp, D.M., Schonberger, M.B., Singer, D.J., Lewitt, P.A. (2004) Early complement activation increases in the brain in some aged normal subjects. *Neurobiol. Aging*, 25, 1001–1007.

[11] Cagnin, A., Brooks, D.J., Kennedy, A.M., Gunn, R.N., Myers, R., Turkheimer, F.E., Jones, T., Banati, R.B. (2001) In-vivo measurement of activated microglia in dementia. *Lancet*, 358, 461–467.

[12] Cagnin, A., Rossor, M., Sampson, E.L., Mackinnon, T., Banati, R.B. (2004) In vivo detection of microglial activation in frontotemporal dementia. *Ann. Neurol*, 56, 894–897.

[13] Aarli, J.A. (2003) Role of cytokines in neurological disorders. *Curr. Med. Chem*, 10, 1931-1937.

[14] Putzu, G.A., Figarella-Branger, D., Bouvier-Labit, C., Liprandi, A., Bianco, N., Pellissier, J.F. (2000) Immunohistochemical localization of cytokines, C5b-9 and ICAM-1 in peripheral nerve of Guillain-Barré syndrome. *J. Neurol. Sci*, 174, 16-21.

[15] Press, R., Deretzi, G., Zou, L.P., Zhu, J., Fredman, P., Lycke, J., Link, H. (2001) IL-10 and IFN-gamma in Guillain-Barré syndrome. Network Members of the Swedish Epidemiological Study Group. *J. Neuroimmunol*, 112, 129-138.

[16] Jander, S., Stoll, G. (2001) Interleukin-18 is induced in acute inflammatory demyelinating polyneuropathy. *J. Neuroimmunol*, 114, 253-258.

[17] Buckley, C., Newsom-Davis, J., Willcox, N., Vincent, A. (2001) Do titin and cytokine antibodies in MG patients predict thymoma or thymoma recurrence? *Neurology*, 57, 1579-1582.

[18] Aarli, J.A. (2000) Rasmussen's encephalitis: a challenge to neuroimmunology. *Curr. Opin. Neurol*, 13, 297-299.

[19] Jankowsky, J.L., Patterson, P.H. (2001) The role of cytokines and growth factors in seizures and their sequelae. *Prog. Neurobiol*, 63, 125-149.

[20] Kerschensteiner, M., Stadelmann, C., Dechant, G., Wekerle, H., Hohlfeld, R. (2003) Neurotrophic cross-talk between the nervous and immune systems: implications for neurological diseases. *Ann. Neurol*, 53, 292-304.

[21] Cowan, W.M. (2001) Viktor Hamburger and Rita Levi-Montalcini: the path to the discovery of nerve growth factor. *Annu. Rev. Neurosci*, 24, 551– 600.

[22] Dalakas, M.C. (2006) B cells in the pathophysiology of autoimmune neurological disorders: a credible therapeutic target. *Pharmacol. Ther*, 112, 57-70.

[23] Anthony, I.C., Crawford, D.H., Bell, J.E. (2003) B lymphocytes in the normal brain: contrasts with HIV-associated lymphoid infiltrates and lymphomas. *Brain*, 126, 1058–1067.

[24] Alter, A., Duddy, M., Hebert, S., Biernacki, K., Prat, A., Antel, J.P., Yong, V.W., Nuttall, R.K., Pennington, C.J., Edwards, D.R., Bar-Or, A. (2003) Determinants of human B cell migration across brain endothelial cells. *J. Immunol*, 170, 4497–4505.

[25] Lucchinetti, C., Bruck, W., Parisi, J., Scheithauer, B., Rodriguez, M., Lassmann, H. (2000) Heterogeneity of multiple sclerosis lesions: implications for the pathogenesis of demyelination. *Ann. Neurol*, 47, 707–717.

[26] Keegan, M., Konig, F., McClelland, R., Brück, W., Morales, Y., Bitsch, A., Panitch, H., Lassmann, H., Weinshenker, B., Rodriguez, M., Parisi, J., Lucchinetti, C.F. (2005) Relation between humoral pathological changes in multiple sclerosis and response to therapeutic plasma exchange. *Lancet*, 366, 579–582.

[27] Qin, Y., Duquette, P., Zhang, Y., Olek, M., Da, R.R., Richardson, J., Antel, J.P., Talbot, P., Cashman, N.R., Tourtellotte, W.W., Wekerle, H., Van Den Noort, S. (2003) Intrathecal B-cell clonal expansion, an early sign of humoral immunity, in the cerebrospinal fluid of patients with clinically isolated syndrome suggestive of multiple sclerosis. *Lab. Invest*, 83, 1081–1088.

[28] Owens, G.P., Ritchie, A.M., Burgoon, M.P., Williamson, R.A., Corboy, J.R., Gilden, D.H. (2003) Single-cell repertoire analysis demonstrates that clonal expansion is a prominent feature of the B cell response in multiple sclerosis cerebrospinal fluid. *J. Immunol*, 171, 2725–2733.

[29] Cepok, S., Jacobsen, M., Schock, S., Omer, B., Jaekel, S., Böddeker, I., Oertel, W.H., Sommer, N., Hemmer, B. (2001) Patterns of cerebrospinal fluid pathology correlate with disease progression in multiple sclerosis. *Brain*, 124, 2169–2176.

[30] Villar, L.M., Sadaba, M.C., Roldan, E., Masjuan, J., González-Porqué, P., Villarrubia, N., Espiño, M., García-Trujillo, J.A., Bootello, A., Alvarez-Cermeño, J.C. (2005) Intrathecal synthesis of oligoclonal IgM against myelin lipids predicts an aggressive disease course in MS. *J. Clin. Invest*, 115, 187–194.

[31] Bar-Or, A., Oliveira, E.M., Anderson, D.E., Krieger, J.I., Duddy, M., O'Connor, K.C., Hafler, D.A. (2001) Immunological memory: contribution of memory B cells expressing costimulatory molecules in the resting state. *J. Immunol*, 167, 5669–5677.

[32] Berger, T., Rubner, P., Schautzer, F., Egg, R., Ulmer, H., Mayringer, I., Dilitz, E., Deisenhammer, F., Reindl, M. (2003) Antimyelin antibodies as a predictor of clinically definite multiple sclerosis after a first demyelinating event. *N. Engl. J. Med*, 349, 139–145.

[33] McLaughlin, K.A., Chitnis, T., Newcombe, J., Franz, B., Kennedy, J., McArdel, S., Kuhle, J., Kappos, L., et al. (2009) Age-dependent B cell autoimmunity to a myelin surface antigen in pediatric multiple sclerosis. *J. Immunol.*, 183, 4067-4076.

[34] Zhou, D., Srivastava, R., Nessler, S., Grummel, V., Sommer, N., Bruck, W., Hartung, H.P., Stadelmann, C., Hemmer, B. (2006) Identification of a pathogenic antibody response to native myelin oligodendrocyte glycoprotein in multiple sclerosis. *Proc. Natl. Acad. Sci. USA*, 103, 19057-19062.

[35] O'Connor, K.C., Appel, H., Bregoli, L., Call, M.E., Catz, I., Chan, J.A., Moore, N.H., Warren, K.G., Wong, S.J., Hafler, D.A., Wucherpfennig, K.W. (2005) Antibodies from inflamed central nervous system tissue recognize myelin oligodendrocyte glycoprotein. *J. Immunol.,* 175, 1974-1982.

[36] Vincent, A., Beeson, D., Lang, B. (2000) Molecular targets for autoimmune and genetic disorders of neuromuscular transmission. *Eur. J. Biochem*, 267, 6717–6728.

[37] Vincent, A., Leite, M.I. (2005) Neuromuscular junction autoimmune disease: muscle specific kinase antibodies and treatments for myasthenia gravis. *Curr. Opin. Neurol*, 18, 519–525.

[38] Buckley, C., Vincent, A. (2005) Autoimmune channelopathies. *Nature Clin. Pract. Neurol*, 1, 22–32.

[39] Vincent, A., Buckley, C., Schott, J. M., Baker, I., Dewar, B.K., Detert, N., Clover, L., Parkinson, A., Bien, C.G., Omer, S., Lang, B., Rossor, M.N., Palace, J. (2004) Potassium channel antibody-associated encephalopathy: a potentially immunotherapy-responsive form of limbic encephalitis. *Brain*, 127, 701–712.

[40] Willison, H. J., Yuki, N. (2002) Peripheral neuropathies and anti-glycolipid antibodies. *Brain*, 125, 2591–2625.

[41] Kuwabara, S. (2004) Guillain-Barré syndrome: epidemiology, pathophysiology and management. *Drugs*, 64, 597–610.

[42] Ogawara, K., Kuwabara, S., Mori, M., Hattori, T., Koga, M., Yuki, N. (2000) Axonal Guillain-Barré syndrome: relation to anti-ganglioside antibodies and Campylobacter jejuni infection in Japan. *Ann. Neurol*, 48, 624–631.

[43] Kieseier, B.C., Kiefer, R., Gold, R., Hemmer, B., Willison, H.J., Hartung, H.P. (2004) Advances in understanding and treatment of immune-mediated disorders of the peripheral nervous system. *Muscle Nerve*, 30, 131–156.

[44] Nobile-Orazio, E. (2001) Multifocal motor neuropathy. *J. Neuroimmunol*, 115, 4–18.

[45] Nobile-Orazio, E. (2004) IgM paraproteinaemic neuropathies. *Curr. Opin. Neurol*, 17, 599–605.

[46] Hendriks, J.J., Teunissen, C.E., de Vries, H.E., Dijkstra, C.D. (2005) Macrophages and neurodegeneration. *Brain Res. Rev*, 48, 185-195.

[47] Kraus, J., Kuehne, B.S., Tofighi, J., Frielinghaus, P., Stolz, E., Blaes, F., Laske, C., Engelhardt, B., Traupe, H., Kaps, M., Oschmann, P. (2002) Serum cytokine levels do not correlate with disease activity and severity assessed by brain MRI in multiple sclerosis. *Acta Neurol. Scand*, 105, 300–308.

[48] Gilgun-Sherki, Y., Melamed, E., Offen, D. (2004) The role of oxidative stress in the pathogenesis of multiple sclerosis: the need for effective antioxidant therapy. *J. Neurol*, 51, 261–268.

[49] Besler, H.T., Comoglu, S. (2003) Lipoprotein oxidation, plasma total antioxidant capacity and homocysteine level in patients with multiple sclerosis. *Nutr. Neurosci*, 5, 189–196.

[50] Touil, T., Deloire-Grassin, M.S., Vital, C., Petry, K.G., Brochet, B. (2001) In vivo damage of CNS myelin and axons induced by peroxynitrite. *Neuro Report*, 12, 3637–3644.

[51] Sarchielli, P., Greco, L., Floridi, A., Gallai, V. (2003) Excitatory amino acids and multiple sclerosis: evidence from cerebrospinal fluid. *Arch Neurol*, 60, 1082–1088.

[52] Geurts, J.J., Wolswijk, G., Bo, L., van der Valk, P., Polman, C.H., Troost, D., Aronica, E. (2003) Altered expression patterns of group I and II metabotropic glutamate receptors in multiple sclerosis. *Brain*, 126, 1755–1766.

[53] Yong, V.W., Power, C., Forsyth, P., Edwards, D.R. (2001) *Nat. Rev. Neurosci*, 2, 502–511.

[54] Bajetto, A., Bonavia, R., Barbero, S., Florio, T., Schettini, G. (2001) Chemokines and their receptors in the central nervous system. *Front Neuroendocrinol*, 22, 147-184.

[55] Simpson, J., Rezaie, P., Newcombe, J., Cuzner, M.L., Male, D., Woodroofe, M.N. (2000) Expression of the beta-chemokine receptors CCR2, CCR3 and CCR5 in multiple sclerosis central nervous system tissue. *J. Neuroimmunol*, 108, 192–200.

[56] Yang, T.Y., Chen, S.C., Leach, M.W., Manfra, D., Homey, B., Wiekowski, M., Sullivan, L., Jenh, C.H., Narula, S.K., Chensue, S.W., Lira, S.A. (2000) Transgenic expression of the chemokine receptor encoded by human herpesvirus 8 induces an angioproliferative disease resembling Kaposi's sarcoma. *J. Exp. Med*, 191, 445–454.

[57] Xia, M., Bacskai, B.J., Knowles, R.B., Qin, S.X., Hyman, B.T. (2000) Expression of the chemokine receptor CXCR3 on neurons and the elevated expression of its ligand IP-10 in reactive astrocytes: in vitro ERK1/2 activation and role in Alzheimer's disease. *J. Neuroimmunol*, 108, 227–235.

[58] Prat, E., Baron, L., Meda, L., Scarpini, E., Galimberti, D., Ardolino, G., Catania, A., Scarlato, G. (2000) The human astrocytoma cell line U373MG produces monocyte chemotactic protein (MCP)-1 upon stimulation with beta-amyloid protein. *Neurosci Lett*, 283, 177–180.

[59] Tracey, K.J. (2007) Physiology and immunology of the cholinergic anti-inflammatory pathway. *J. Clin. Invest.*, 117, 289–296.

[60] Borovikova, L.V., Ivanova, S., Zhang, M., Yang, H., Botchkina, G.I., Watkins, L.R., Wang, H., Abumrad, N., Eaton, J.W., Tracey, K.J. (2000) Vagus nerve stimulation attenuates the systemic inflammatory response to endotoxin. *Nature*, 405, 458–462.

[61] Mioni, C., Bazzani, C., Giuliani, D., Altavilla, D., Leone, S., Ferrari, A., Minutoli, L., Bitto, A., Marini, H., Zaffe, D., Botticelli, A.R., Iannone, A., Tomasi, A., Bigiani, A., Bertolini, A., Squadrito, F., Guarini, S. (2005) Activation of an efferent cholinergic pathway produces strong protection against myocardial ischemia/reperfusion injury in rats. *Crit. Care Med*, 33, 2621–2628.

[62] Altavilla, D., Guarini, S., Bitto, A., Mioni, C., Giuliani, D., Bigiani, A., Squadrito, G., Minutoli, L., Venuti, F.S., Messineo, F., De Meo, V., Bazzani, C., Squadrito, F. (2006) Activation of the cholinergic anti-inflammatory pathway reduces NF-kappab activation, blunts TNF-alpha production, and protects againts splanchic artery occlusion shock. *Shock*, 25, 500–506.

[63] Guarini, S., Altavilla, D., Cainazzo, M.M., Giuliani, D., Bigiani, A., Marini, H., Squadrito, G., Minutoli, L., Bertolini, A., Marini, R., Adamo, E.B., Venuti, F.S., Squadrito, F. (2003) Efferent vagal fibre stimulation blunts nuclear factor-kappaB activation and protects against hypovolemic hemorrhagic shock. *Circulation*, 107, 1189–1194.

[64] de Jonge, W.J., van der Zanden, E.P., The FO, Bijlsma, M.F., van Westerloo, D.J., Bennink, R.J., Berthoud, H.R., Uematsu, S., Akira, S., van den Wijngaard, R.M., Boeckxstaens, G.E. (2005) Stimulation of the vagus nerve attenuates macrophage activation by activating the Jak2-STAT3 signaling pathway. *Nat. Immunol*, 6, 844–851.

[65] Borovikova, L.V., Ivanova, S., Nardi, D., Zhang, M., Yang, H., Ombrellino, M., Tracey, K.J. (2000) Role of vagus nerve signaling in CNI-1493-mediated suppression of acute inflammation. *Auton. Neurosci*, 85, 141–147.

[66] van Westerloo, D.J., Giebelen, I.A., Florquin, S., Bruno, M.J., Larosa, G.J., Ulloa, L., Tracey, K.J., van der Poll, T. (2006) The vagus nerve and nicotinic receptors modulate experimental pancreatitis severity in mice. *Gastroenterology*, 130, 1822–1830.

[67] Saeed, R.W., Varma, S., Peng-Nemeroff, T., Sherry, B., Balakhaneh, D., Huston, J., Tracey, K.J., Al-Abed, Y., Metz, C.N. (2005) Cholinergic stimulation blocks endothelial cell activation and leukocyte recruitment during inflammation. *J. Exp. Med*, 201, 1113–1123.

[68] Wang, H., Yu, M., Ochani, M., et al. (2003) *Nature*, 421, 384–388.

[69] Rosas-Ballina M, Tracey KJ. (2009) Cholinergic control of inflammation. *J. Intern. Med*, 265, 663-679.

[70] Tracey, K.J. (2007) Physiology and immunology of the cholinergic antiinflammatory pathway. *J. Clin. Invest*, 117, 289-296.

[71] Bach, J.F. (2003) Regulatory T cells under scrutiny. *Nat. Rev. Immunol*, 3, 189-198.

[72] Lassmann, H., Brück, W., Lucchinetti, C. (2001) Heterogeneity of multiple sclerosis pathogenesis: implications for diagnosis and therapy. *Trends Mol. Med*, 7, 115-121.

[73] Muraro, P.A., Kalbus, M., Afshar, G., et al. (2002) T cell response to 2',3'-cyclic nucleotide 3'-phosphodiesterase (CNPase) in multiple sclerosis patients. *J. Neuroimmunol*, 130, 233-242.

[74] Antel, J., Birnbaum, G., Hartung, H-P., et al., Clinical Neuroimmunology, 2nd Edition Oxford University Press The immunology of multiple sclerosis. (2005); pp 185-194.

[75] Cavaletti, G. (2006) Current status and future prospective of immunointervention in multiple sclerosis. *Curr. Med. Chem*, 13, 2329-2343.

[76] Edan, G., Morrissey, S., Le Page, E. (2004) Rationale for the use of mitoxantrone in multiple sclerosis. *J. Neurol.. Sci*, 223, 35-39.

[77] Martinelli, B.F., Rovaris, M., et al. (2005) Cochrane Database Syst. Rev., 19, CD002127.

[78] Gonsette, R.E., Dubois, B. (2004) Pixantrone (BBR2778): a new immunosuppressant in multiple sclerosis with a low cardiotoxicity. *J. Neurol. Sci*, 223, 81-86.

[79] Fernández, O., Fernández, V., De Ramón, E. (2004) Azathioprine and methotrexate in multiple sclerosis. *J. Neurol. Sci*, 223, 29-34.

[80] Reggio, E., Nicoletti, A., Fiorilla, T., Politi, G., Reggio, A., Patti, F. (2005) The combination of cyclophosphamide plus interferon beta as rescue therapy could be used to treat relapsing-remitting multiple sclerosis patients-- twenty-four months follow-up. *J. Neurol*, 252, 1255-1261.

[81] Gray, O., McDonnell, G.V., Forbes, R.B. (2004) Cochrane Database Syst. Rev., CD003208.

[82] Calabresi, P.A., Wilterdink, J.L., Rogg, J.M., Mills, P., Webb, A., Whartenbay, K.E. (2002), An open-label trial of combination therapy with interferon beta-1a and oral methotrexate in MS. *Neurology*, 58, 314-317.

[83] Frohman, E.M., Brannon, K., Racke, M.K., Hawker, K. (2004) Mycophenolate mofetil in multiple sclerosis. *Clin. Neuropharmacol*, 27, 80-83.

[84] Gray, O., McDonnell, G.V., Forbes, R.B., (2003), Cochrane Database Syst. Rev., CD002936.

[85] Achiron, A., Kishner, I., Dolev, M., Stern Y, Dulitzky M, Schiff E, Achiron R. (2004) Effect of intravenous immunoglobulin treatment on pregnancy and postpartum-related relapses in multiple sclerosis. *J. Neurol*, 251, 1133-1137.

[86] Sellebjerg, F., Barnes, D., Filippini, G., Midgard, R., Montalban, X., Rieckmann, P., Selmaj, K., Visser, L.H., Sørensen, P.S.; EFNS Task Force on Treatment of Multiple Sclerosis Relapses. (2005) EFNS guideline on treatment of multiple sclerosis relapses: report of an EFNS task force on treatment of multiple sclerosis relapses. *Eur. J. Neurol*, 12, 939-946.

[87] Ruprecht, K., Klinker, E., Dintelmann, T., Rieckmann, P., Gold, R. (2004) Plasma exchange for severe optic neuritis: treatment of 10 patients. *Neurology*, 63, 1081-1083.

[88] Havrdova, E. (2005) Aggressive multiple sclerosis-is there a role for stem cell transplantation? *J. Neurol*, 252, iii34-37.

[89] Blanco, Y., Saiz, A., Carreras, E., Graus, F. (2005) Autologous haematopoietic-stem-cell transplantation for multiple sclerosis. *Lancet Neurol*, 4, 54-63.

[90] Comi, G., Kappos, L., Clanet, M., Ebers, G., Fassas, A., Fazekas, F., Filippi, M., Hartung, H.P., Hertenstein, B., Karussis, D., Martino, G., Tyndall, A., van der Meché, F.G. (2000) Guidelines for autologous blood and marrow stem cell transplantation in multiple sclerosis: a consensus report written on behalf of the European Group for Blood and Marrow Transplantation and the European Charcot Foundation. BMT-MS Study Group. *J. Neurol*, 247, 376-382.

[91] Adorini, L. (2004) Immunotherapeutic approaches in multiple sclerosis. *J. Neurol. Sci*, 223, 13-24.

[92] Vernino, S. (2007) Autoimmune and paraneoplastic channelopathies. *Neurotherapeutics*, 4, 305-314.

[93] Vernino, S., Low, P.A., Fealey, R.D., Stewart, J.D., Farrugia, G., Lennon, V.A. (2000) Autoantibodies to ganglionic acetylcholine receptors in autoimmune autonomic neuropathies. *N. Engl. J. Med*, 343, 847–855.

[94] Goldstein, D., Holmes, C., Dendi, R., Li, S.T., Brentzel, S., Vernino, S. (2002) Pandysautonomia associated with impaired ganglionic neurotransmission and circulating antibody to the neuronal nicotinic receptor. *Clin. Auton. Res*, 12, 281–285.

[95] Schroeder, C., Vernino, S., Birkenfeld, A.L., Tank, J., Heusser, K., Lipp, A., Benter, T., Lindschau, C., Kettritz, R., Luft, F.C., Jordan, J. (2005) Plasma exchange for primary autoimmune autonomic failure. *N. Engl. J. Med*, 353, 1585–1590.

[96] Rajakulendran, S., Schorge, S., Kullmann, D.M., Hanna, M.G. (2007) Episodic ataxia type 1: a neuronal potassium channelopathy. *Neurotherapeutics*, 4, 258-266.

[97] Hart, I.K., Maddison, P., Newsom-Davis, J., Vincent, A., Mills, K.R. (2002) Phenotypic variants of autoimmune peripheral nerve hyperexcitability. *Brain*, 125, 1887–1895.

[98] Vernino, S., Lennon, V.A. (2002) Phenotypic variants of autoimmune peripheral nerve hyperexcitability. *Muscle Nerve*, 26, 702–707.

[99] Kleopa, K.A., Elman, L.B., Lang, B., Vincent, A., Scherer, S.S. (2006) Neuromyotonia and limbic encephalitis sera target mature Shaker-type K+ channels: subunit specificity correlates with clinical manifestations. *Brain*, 129, 1570–1584.

[100] Thieben, M.J., Lennon, V.A., Boeve, B.F., et al. (2004) Neuromyotonia and limbic encephalitis sera target mature Shaker-type K+ channels: subunit specificity correlates with clinical manifestations. *Neurology*, 62, 1177–1182.

[101] Watson, R., Jepson, J.E., Bermudez, I., Alexander, S., Hart, Y., McKnight, K., Roubertie, A., Fecto, F., Valmier, J., Sattelle, D.B., Beeson, D., Vincent, A., Lang, B. (2005) Alpha7-acetylcholine receptor antibodies in two patients with Rasmussen encephalitis. *Neurology*, 65, 1802–1804.

[102] Graber, D.J., Levy, M., Kerr, D., Wade, WF. (2008) Neuromyelitis optica pathogenesis and aquaporin 4. *J. Neuroinflammation*, 5, 22.

[103] Prins, R.M., Liau, L.M. (2003) Immunology and immunotherapy in neurosurgical disease. *Neurosurgery*, 53, 144-152.

[104] Graf, M.R., Prins, R.M., Merchant, R.E. (2001) IL-6 secretion by a rat T9 glioma clone induces a neutrophil-dependent antitumor response with resultant cellular, antiglioma immunity. *J. Immunol*, 166, 121–129.

[105] Jung, G., Brandl, M., Eisner, W., Fraunberger, P., Reifenberger, G., Schlegel, U., Wiestler, O.D., Reulen, H.J., Wilmanns, W. (2001) Local immunotherapy of glioma patients with a combination of 2 bispecific antibody fragments and resting autologous lymphocytes: evidence for in situ t-cell activation and therapeutic efficacy. *Int. J. Cancer*, 91, 225–230.

[106] Reardon, D.A., Akabani, G., Coleman, R.E., Friedman, A.H., Friedman, H.S., Herndon, J.E. 2nd, Cokgor, I., McLendon, R.E., Pegram, C.N., Provenzale, J.M., Quinn, J.A., Rich, J.N., Regalado, L.V., Sampson, J.H., Shafman, T.D., Wikstrand, C.J., Wong, T.Z., Zhao, X.G., Zalutsky, M.R., Bigner, D.D. (2002) Phase II trial of murine (131)I-labeled antitenascin monoclonal antibody 81C6 administered into surgically created resection cavities of patients with newly diagnosed malignant gliomas. *J. Clin. Oncol*, 20, 1389–1397.

[107] Pardoll, D.M. (2002) Spinning molecular immunology into successful immunotherapy. *Nat. Rev. Immunol*, 2, 227–238.

[108] de Beukelaar, J.W., Sillevis Smitt, P.A. (2006) Managing paraneoplastic neurological disorders. *Oncologist*, 11, 292-305.

[109] Graus, F., Keime-Guibert, F., Rene, R., Benyahia, B., Ribalta, T., Ascaso, C., Escaramis, G., Delattre, J.Y. (2001) Anti-Hu-associated paraneoplastic encephalo myelitis: analysis of 200 patients. *Brain*, 124, 1138–1148.

[110] Sillevis Smitt, P., Grefkens, J., De Leeuw, B., van den Bent, M., van Putten, W., Hooijkaas, H., Vecht, C. (2002) Survival and outcome in 73 anti-Hu positive patients with paraneoplastic encephalomyelitis/sensory neuronopathy. *J. Neurol*, 249, 745–753.

[111] Keime-Guibert, F., Graus, F., Fleury, A., René, R., Honnorat, J., Broet, P., Delattre, J.Y. (2000) Treatment of paraneoplastic neurological syndromes with antineuronal antibodies (Anti-Hu, anti-Yo) with a combination of immunoglobulins, cyclophosphamide, and methylprednisolone. *J. Neurol. Neurosurg. Psychiatry*, 68, 479–482.

[112] Foster AR, Caplan JP. (2009) Paraneoplastic limbic encephalitis. *Psychosomatics*, 50, 108-113.

[113] Shams'ili, S., de Beukelaar, J., Gratama, J.W., Hooijkaas, H., van den Bent, M., van 't Veer, M., Sillevis Smitt, P. (2006) An uncontrolled trial of rituximab for antibody associated paraneoplastic neurological syndromes. *J. Neurol*, 253, 16–20.

[114] Wirtz, P.W., Sillevis Smitt, P.A., Hoff, J.I., Hoff, J.I., de Leeuw, B., Lammers, G.J., van Duinen, S.G., Verschuuren, J.J. (2002) Anti-Ri antibody positive opsoclonus-myoclonus in a male patient with breast carcinoma. *J. Neurol*, 249, 1710-1712.

[115] Visser, L.H., Beekman, R., Tijssen, C.C., Uitdehaag, B.M., Lee, M.L., Movig, K.L., Lenderink, A.W. (2004) A randomized, double-blind, placebo-controlled pilot study of i.v. immune globulins in combination with i.v. methylprednisolone in the treatment of relapses in patients with MS. *Mult. Scler*, 10, 89–91.

[116] Achiron, A., Kishner, I., Sarova-Pinhas, I., Raz, H., Faibel, M., Stern, Y., Lavie, M., Gurevich, M., Dolev, M., Magalashvili, D., Barak, Y. (2004) Intravenous immunoglobulin treatment following the first demyelinating event suggestive of multiple sclerosis: a randomized, double-blind, placebo-controlled trial. *Arch Neurol*, 61, 1515–1520.

[117] Linker, R.A., Gold, R. (2008) Use of intravenous immunoglobulin and plasma exchange in neurological disease. *Curr. Opin. Neurol*, 21, 358-365.

[118] van Koningsveld, R., Schmitz, P.I., Meche, F.G., Visser, L.H., Meulstee, J., van Doorn, P.A.; Dutch GBS study group. (2004) Effect of methylprednisolone when added to standard treatment with intravenous immunoglobulin for Guillain-Barré syndrome: randomised trial. *Lancet*, 363, 192–196.

[119] Mori, M., Kuwabara, S., Fukutake, T., Hattori, T. (2007) Intravenous immunoglobulin therapy for Miller Fisher syndrome. *Neurology*, 68, 1144–1146.

[120] Hughes, R.A., Donofrio, P., Bril, V., Dalakas, M.C., Deng, C., Hanna, K., Hartung, H.P., Latov, N., Merkies, I.S., van Doorn, P.A; ICE Study Group. (2008) Intravenous immune globulin (10% caprylate-chromatography purified) for the treatment of chronic inflammatory demyelinating polyradiculoneuropathy (ICE study): a randomised placebo-controlled trial. *Lancet Neurol*, 7, 136–144.

[121] Sharma, K.R., Cross, J., Ayyar, D.R., Martinez-Arizala, A., Bradley, W.G. (2002) Diabetic demyelinating polyneuropathy responsive to intravenous immunoglobulin therapy. *Arch Neurol*, 59, 751–757.

[122] Levy, Y., Uziel, Y., Zandman, G.G., Amital, H., Sherer, Y., Langevitz, P., Goldman, B., Shoenfeld, Y. (2003) Intravenous immunoglobulins in peripheral neuropathy associated with vasculitis. *Ann. Rheum. Dis*, 62, 1221-1223.

[123] Van Schaik, I., van den Berg, L.H., De, H.R., et al. (2005) Cochrane Database Syst. Rev., CD004429.

[124] Zinman, L., Ng, E., Bril, V. (2007) IV immunoglobulin in patients with myasthenia gravis: a randomized controlled trial. *Neurology*, 68, 837–841.

[125] Trikha, I., Singh, S., Goyal, V., Shukla, G., Bhasin, R., Behari, M. (2007) Comparative efficacy of low dose, daily versus alternate day plasma exchange in severe myasthenia gravis: a randomised trial. *J. Neurol*, 254, 989–995.

[126] Walter, M.C., Lochmuller, H., Toepfer, M., Schlotter, B., Reilich, P., Schröder, M., Müller-Felber, W., Pongratz, D. (2000) High-dose immunoglobulin therapy in sporadic inclusion body myositis: a double-blind, placebo-controlled study. *J. Neurol*, 247, 22–28.

[127] Szczepiorkowski, Z.M., Bandarenko, N., Kim, H.C., Linenberger, M.L., Marques, M.B., Sarode, R., Schwartz, J., Shaz, B.H., Weinstein, R., Wirk, A., Winters, J.L.; American Society for Apheresis; Apheresis Applications Committee of the American Society for Apheresis. (2007) Guidelines on the use of therapeutic apheresis in clinical practice: evidence-based approach from the Apheresis Applications Committee of the American Society for Apheresis. *J. Clin. Apher*, 22, 106–175.

[128] Basic-Jukic, N., Kes, P., Glavasa-Boras, S., Brunetta, B., Bubic-Filipi, L., Puretic, Z. (2005) Complications of therapeutic plasma exchange: experience with 4857 treatments. *Ther. Apher. Dial*, 9, 391–395.
[129] Weinstein, R. (2000) Therapeutic apheresis in neurological disorders. *J. Clin. Apher*, 15, 74–128.
[130] McLeod, B.C., Therapeutic plasma exchange in neurologic disorders. In: McLeod BC, Price TH, Weinstein R, editors. Apheresis: principles and practice. Bethasda, MD: AABB Press; (2003). p. 321–44.
[131] Said, G. (2006) Chronic inflammatory demyelinating polyneuropathy. *Neuromuscul. Disord*, 16, 293–303.
[132] Hehmann, H.C., Hartung, H.P., Hetzel, G.R., Stüve, O., Kieseier, B.C. (2006) Plasma exchange in neuroimmunological disorders: part 2. Treatment of neuromuscular disorders. *Arch Neurol*, 63, 1066–1071.
[133] Raphael, J.C., Chevret, S., Hughes, R.A.C., et al. (2002) Cochrane Database Syst. Rev., (2), CD001798.
[134] Gajdos, P. (2002) Cochrane Database Syst. Rev., (4), CD002275.
[135] Shah, A.K., Tselis, A., Mason, B. (2000) Acute disseminated encephalomyelitis in a pregnant woman successfully treated with plasmapheresis. *J. Neurol. Sci*, 174, 147–151.
[136] Keegan, M., Pineda, A.A., McClelland, R.L., Darby, C.H., Rodriguez, M., Weinshenker, B.G. (2002) Plasma exchange for severe attacks of CNS demyelination: predictors of response. *Neurology*, 58, 143–146.
[137] Colasanti, T., Delunardo, F., Margutti, P., Vacirca, D., Piro, E., Siracusano, A., Ortona, E. (2009) Autoantibodies involved in neuropsychiatric manifestations associated with systemic lupus erythematosus. *J. Neuroimmunol*, 212, 3-9.
[138] Carney, R.M., Blumenthal, J.A., Catellier, D., Freedland, K.E., Berkman, L.F., Watkins, L.L., Czajkowski, S.M., Hayano, J., Jaffe, A.S. (2003) Depression as a risk factor for mortality after acute myocardial infarction. *Am. J. Cardiol*, 92, 1277-1281.
[139] Ramasawmy, R., Faé, K.C., Spina, G., Victora, G.D., Tanaka, A.C., Palácios, S.A., Hounie, A.G., Miguel, E.C., Oshiro, S.E., Goldberg, A.C., Kalil, J., Guilherme, L. (2007) Association of polymorphisms within the promoter region of the tumor necrosis factor-alpha with clinical outcomes of rheumatic fever. *Mol. Immunol* 44, 1873-1878.
[140] Sanders, V.M., Kohm, A.P. (2002) Sympathetic nervous system interaction with the immune system. *Int. Rev. Neurobiol*, 52, 17-41.
[141] Marques-Deak, A., Cizza, G., Sternberg, E. (2005) Brain-immune interactions and disease susceptibility. *Mol. Psychiatry*, 10, 239-250.
[142] Tracey, K.J. (2002) The inflammatory reflex. *Nature*, 420, 853-859.
[143] Chaplin, D.D. (2003) The effect of neonatal BCG vaccination on atopy and asthma at age 7 to 14 years: an historical cohort study in a community with a very low prevalence of tuberculosis infection and a high prevalence of atopic disease. *J. Allergy Clin. Immunol*, 111, 541-549.
[144] Rocha, B., Tanchot, C. (2004) Towards a cellular definition of CD8+ T-cell memory: the role of CD4+ T-cell help in CD8+ T-cell responses. *Curr. Opin. Immunol*, 16, 259-263.
[145] Steinman, L. (2004) Elaborate interactions between the immune and nervous systems. *Nat. Immunol*, 5, 575-581.

[146] Ramaglia, V., Baas, F. (2009) Innate immunity in the nervous system. *Prog. Brain Res*, 175, 95-123.
[147] Kang, S.S., McGavern, D.B. (2009) Inflammation on the mind: visualizing immunity in the central nervous system. *Curr. Top Microbiol. Immunol*, 334, 227-263.
[148] Rosas-Ballina, M., Tracey, K.J. (2009) Cholinergic control of inflammation. *J. Intern. Med*, 265, 663-679.
[149] Sapolsky, R.M., Romero, L.M., Munck, A.U. (2000) How do glucocorticoids influence stress responses? Integrating permissive, suppressive, stimulatory, and preparative actions. *Endocr. Rev*, 21, 55-89.
[150] Del Rey, A., Besedovsky, H.O., Sorkin, E., da Prada, M., Arrenbrecht, S. (1981) Immunoregulation mediated by the sympathetic nervous system, II. *Cell Immunol*, 63, 329-334.
[151] Felten, D.L., Felten, S.Y., Bellinger, D.L., Carlson, S.L., Ackerman, K.D., Madden, K.S., Olschowki, J.A., Livnat, S. (1987) Noradrenergic sympathetic neural interactions with the immune system: structure and function. *Immunol. Rev*, 100, 225-260.
[152] Elenkov, I.J., Wilder, R.L., Chrousos, G.P., Vizi, E.S. (2000) The sympathetic nerve--an integrative interface between two supersystems: the brain and the immune system. *Pharmacol. Rev*, 52, 595-638.
[153] Swanson, M.A., Lee, W.T., Sanders, V.M. (2001) IFN-gamma production by Th1 cells generated from naive CD4+ T cells exposed to norepinephrine. *J. Immunol*, 166, 232-240.
[154] De Coupade, C., Gear, R.W., Dazin, P.F., Sroussi HY, Green PG, Levine JD. (2004) Beta 2-adrenergic receptor regulation of human neutrophil function is sexually dimorphic. *Br. J. Pharmacol*, 143, 1033-1041.
[155] Leonard, B.E., Song, C. (1999) Stress, depression, and the role of cytokines. *Adv. Exp. Med. Biol*, 461, 251-265.
[156] O'Connor, T.M., O'Halloran, D.J., Shanahan, F. (2000) The stress response and the hypothalamic-pituitary-adrenal axis: from molecule to melancholia. *QJM*, 93, 323-333.
[157] McGeer, P.L., McGeer, E.G. (1995) The inflammatory response system of brain: implications for therapy of Alzheimer and other neurodegenerative diseases. *Brain Res. Brain Res. Rev*, 21, 195-218.
[158] Anisman, H., Hayley, S., Turrin, N., Merali, Z. (2002) Cytokines as a stressor: implications for depressive illness. *Int. J. Neuropsychopharmacol*, 5, 357-373.
[159] Brebner, K,, Hayley, S., Zacharko, R., Merali, Z., Anisman, H. (2000) Synergistic effects of interleukin-1beta, interleukin-6, and tumor necrosis factor-alpha: central monoamine, corticosterone, and behavioral variations. *Neuropsychopharmacology*, 22, 566-580.
[160] Dantzer, R., Kelley, K.W. (2007) Twenty years of research on cytokine-induced sickness behavior. *Brain Behav. Immun*, 21, 153-160.
[161] Capuron, L., Ravaud, A., Dantzer, R. (2000) Early depressive symptoms in cancer patients receiving interleukin 2 and/or interferon alfa-2b therapy. *J. Clin. Oncol*, 18, 2143-2151.
[162] Raisons, C.L., Capuron, L., Miller, A.H. (2006) Cytokines sing the blues: inflammation and the pathogenesis of depression. *Trends Immunol*, 27, 24-31.
[163] Capuron, L,, Miller, A.H. (2004) Cytokines and psychopathology: lessons from interferon-alpha. *Biol. Psychiatry*, 56,819-824.

[164] Capuron, L., Ravaud, A. (1999) Prediction of the depressive effects of interferon alfa therapy by the patient's initial affective state. *N. Engl. J. Med*, 340, 1370.

[165] Sutcigil, L., Oktenli, C., Musabak, U., Bozkurt, A., Cansever, A., Uzun, O., Sanisoglu, S.Y., Yesilova, Z., Ozmenler, N., Ozsahin, A., Sengul, A. (2007) Pro- and anti-inflammatory cytokine balance in major depression: effect of sertraline therapy. *Clin. Dev. Immunol.*, 76396, 1-6.

[166] Felten, D.L., Felten, S.Y., Carlson, S.L, Olschowka, J.A., Livnat, S. (1985) Noradrenergic and peptidergic innervation of lymphoid tissue. *J. Immunol*, 135, 755-765.

[167] Guerrero, J.M., Reiter, R.J. (1992) A brief survey of pineal gland-immune system interrelationships. *Endocr. Res*, 18, 91-113.

[168] Ericsson, A., Kovács, K.J., Sawchenko, P.E. (1994) A functional anatomical analysis of central pathways subserving the effects of interleukin-1 on stress-related neuroendocrine neurons. *J. Neurosci*, 14, 897-913.

[169] Dantzer, R. (2001) Cytokine-induced sickness behavior: mechanisms and implications. *Ann. N. Y. Acad. Sci*, 933, 222-234.

[170] Hansen, M.K., O'Connor, K.A., Goehler, L.E., Watkins, L.R., Maier, S.F. (2001) The contribution of the vagus nerve in interleukin-1beta-induced fever is dependent on dose. *Am. J. Physiol. Regul. Integr. Comp. Physiol*, 280, 929-934.

[171] Luheshi, G.N., Bluthé, R.M., Rushforth, D., Mulcahy, N., Konsman, J.P., Goldbach, M., Dantzer, R. (2000) Vagotomy attenuates the behavioural but not the pyrogenic effects of interleukin-1 in rats. *Auton. Neurosci*, 85, 127-132.

[172] Yang, Z.J., Rao, Z.R., Ju, G. (2000) Evidence for the medullary visceral zone as a neural station of neuroimmunomodulation. *Neurosci. Res*, 38, 237-247.

[173] Borovikova, L.V., Ivanova, S., Zhang, M., Yang, H., Botchkina, G.I., Watkins, L.R., Wang, H., Abumrad, N., Eaton, J.W., Tracey, K.J. (2000) Vagus nerve stimulation attenuates the systemic inflammatory response to endotoxin. *Nature*, 405, 458-462.

[174] Wang, H., Yu, M., Ochani, M., Amella, C.A., Tanovic, M., Susarla, S., Li, J.H., Wang, H., Yang, H., Ulloa, L., Al-Abed, Y., Czura, C.J., Tracey, K.J. (2003) Nicotinic acetylcholine receptor alpha7 subunit is an essential regulator of inflammation. *Nature*, 421, 384-388.

[175] Banks, W.A. (2004) Neuroimmune networks and communication pathways: the importance of location. *Brain Behav. Immun*, 18, 120-122.

[176] Eskandari, F., Webster, J.I., Sternberg, E.M. (2003) Neural immune pathways and their connection to inflammatory diseases. *Arthritis Res. Ther*, 5, 251-265.

[177] Vilcek, J. (2003) Novel interferons. *Nat. Immunol*, 4, 8-9.

[178] Silverman, M.N., Pearce, B.D., Biron, C.A., Miller, A.H. (2005) Immune modulation of the hypothalamic-pituitary-adrenal (HPA) axis during viral infection. *Viral Immunol*, 18, 41-78.

[179] Yu, Y.W., Chen, T.J., Hong, C.J., Chen, H.M., Tsai, S.J. (2003) Association study of the interleukin-1 beta (C-511T) genetic polymorphism with major depressive disorder, associated symptomatology, and antidepressant response. *Neuropsychopharmacology*, 28, 1182-1185.

[180] Jun, T.Y., Pae, C.U., Chae, J.H., Bahk, W.M., Kim, K.S., Pyo, C.W., Han, H. (2003) Tumor necrosis factor-beta gene polymorphism may not be associated with major depressive disorder in the Korean population. *Psychiatry Clin. Neurosci*, 57, 31-35.

[181] Thomas, A.J., Davis, S., Morris, C., Jackson, E., Harrison, R., O'Brien, J.T. (2005) Increase in interleukin-1beta in late-life depression. *Am. J. Psychiatry*, 162, 175-177.

[182] Marques-Deak, A.H., Neto, F.L., Dominguez, W.V., Solis, A.C., Kurcgant, D., Sato, F., Ross, J.M., Prado, E.B. (2007) Cytokine profiles in women with different subtypes of major depressive disorder. *J. Psychiatr Res*, 41, 152-159.

[183] Alesci, S., Martinez, P.E., Kelkar, S., Ilias, I., Ronsaville, D.S., Listwak, S.J., Ayala, A.R., Licinio, J., Gold, H.K., Kling, M.A., Chrousos, G.P., Gold, P.W. (2005) Major depression is associated with significant diurnal elevations in plasma interleukin-6 levels, a shift of its circadian rhythm, and loss of physiological complexity in its secretion: clinical implications. *J. Clin. Endocrinol. Metab*, 90, 2522-2530.

[184] O'Brien, S.M., Scully, P., Fitzgerald, P., Scott, L.V., Dinan, T.G. (2007) Plasma cytokine profiles in depressed patients who fail to respond to selective serotonin reuptake inhibitor therapy. *J. Psychiatr. Res*, 41, 326-331.

[185] Cizza, G., Ravn, P., Chrousos, G.P., Gold, P.W. (2001) Depression: a major, unrecognized risk factor for osteoporosis? *Trends Endocrinol. Metab*, 12, 198-203.

[186] Kenis, G., Maes, M. (2002) Effects of antidepressants on the production of cytokines. *Int. J. Neuropsychopharmacol*, 5, 401-412.

[187] Kaestner, F., Hettich, M., Peters, M., Sibrowski, W., Hetzel, G., Ponath, G., Arolt, V., Cassens, U., Rothermundt, M. (2005) Different activation patterns of proinflammatory cytokines in melancholic and non-melancholic major depression are associated with HPA axis activity. *J. Affect Disord*, 87, 305-311.

[188] Schlatter, J., Ortuño, F., Cervera-Enguix, S. (2004) Lymphocyte subsets and lymphokine production in patients with melancholic versus nonmelancholic depression. *Psychiatry Res*, 128, 259-265.

[189] O'Connor, K.A., Johnson, J.D., Hansen, M.K., Wieseler Frank, J.L., Maksimova, E., Watkins, L.R., Maier, S.F. (2003) Peripheral and central proinflammatory cytokine response to a severe acute stressor. *Brain Res*, 991, 123-132.

[190] Segerstrom, S.C., Miller, G.E. (2004) Psychological stress and the human immune system: a meta-analytic study of 30 years of inquiry. *Psychol Bull*, 130, 601-630.

[191] Dhabhar FS. (2009) Enhancing versus suppressive effects of stress on immune function: implications for immunoprotection and immunopathology. *Neuroimmunomodulation*, 16, 300-317.

[192] Amkraut, A.A., Solomon, G.F., Kraemer, H.C. (1971) Stress, early experience and adjuvant-induced arthritis in the rat. *Psychosom. Med*, 33, 203-214.

[193] Bartrop, R.W., Luckhurst, E., Lazarus, L., Kiloh, L.G., Penny, R. (1977) Depressed lymphocyte function after bereavement. *Lancet*, 1, 834-836.

[194] Glaser, R., Kiecolt-Glaser, J.K. (2005) Stress-induced immune dysfunction: implications for health. *Nat. Rev. Immunol*, 5, 243-251.

[195] Vedhara, K., Cox, N.K., Wilcock, G.K., Perks, P., Hunt, M., Anderson, S., Lightman, S.L., Shanks, N.M. (1999) Chronic stress in elderly carers of dementia patients and antibody response to influenza vaccination. *Lancet*, 353, 627-631.

[196] Cohen, S., Doyle, W.J., Skoner, D.P. (1999) Psychological stress, cytokine production, and severity of upper respiratory illness. *Psychosom. Med*, 61, 175-180.

[197] Schneiderman, N., Antoni, M.H., Fletcher, M.A., Ironson, G., Klimas, N., Kumar, M., LaPerriere, A. (1993) Stress, endocrine responses, immunity and HIV-1 spectrum disease. *Adv. Exp. Med. Biol*, 335, 225-234.

[198] Sheridan, J.F., Padgett, D.A., Avitsur, R., Wiseman, G.A., Sebo, T.J., Grant, C.S. (2004) Sensitivity and utility of parathyroid scintigraphy in patients with primary versus secondary and tertiary hyperparathyroidism. *World J. Surg*, 28, 327-332.

[199] Miller, G.E., Cohen, S., Pressman, S., Barkin, A., Rabin, B.S., Treanor, J.J. (2004) Psychological stress and antibody response to influenza vaccination: when is the critical period for stress, and how does it get inside the body? *Psychosom. Med*, 66, 215-223.

[200] Kiecolt-Glaser, J.K., Glaser, R., Gravenstein, S., Malarkey, W.B., Sheridan, J. (1996) Chronic stress alters the immune response to influenza virus vaccine in older adults. *Proc. Natl. Acad. Sci. USA*, 93, 3043.

[201] Castellani, M.L., Bhattacharya, K., Tagen, M., Kempuraj, D., Perrella, A., De Lutiis, M., Boucher, W., Conti, P., Theoharides, T.C., Cerulli, G., Salini, V., Neri, G. (2007) Anti-chemokine therapy for inflammatory diseases. *Int. J. Immunopathol. Pharmacol*, 20, 447-453.

[202] Witek-Janusek, L., Gabram, S., Mathews, H.L. (2007) Psychologic stress, reduced NK cell activity, and cytokine dysregulation in women experiencing diagnostic breast biopsy. *Psychoneuroendocrinology*, 32, 22-35.

[203] Gerra, G., Monti, D., Panerai, A.E., Sacerdote, P., Anderlini, R., Avanzini, P., Zaimovic, A., Brambilla, F., Franceschi, C. (2003) Long-term immune-endocrine effects of bereavement: relationships with anxiety levels and mood. *Psychiatry Res*, 121, 145-158.

[204] Leserman, J., Petitto, J.M., Golden, R.N., Gaynes, B.N., Gu, H., Perkins, D.O., Silva, S.G., Folds, J.D., Evans, D.L. (2000) Impact of stressful life events, depression, social support, coping, and cortisol on progression to AIDS. *Am. J. Psychiatry*, 157, 1221-1228.

[205] Maes, M., Song, C., Lin, A., De Jongh, R., Van Gastel, A., Kenis, G., Bosmans, E., De Meester, I., Benoy, I., Neels, H., Demedts, P., Janca, A., Scharpé, S., Smith, R.S. (1998) The effects of psychological stress on humans: increased production of pro-inflammatory cytokines and a Th1-like response in stress-induced anxiety. *Cytokine*, 10, 313-318.

[206] Appels, A., Kop, W.J., Schouten, E. (2000) The nature of the depressive symptomatology preceding myocardial infarction. *Behav. Med*, 26, 86-89.

[207] Pradhan, A.D., Manson, J.E., Rifai, N., Buring, J.E., Ridker, P.M. (2001) C-reactive protein, interleukin 6, and risk of developing type 2 diabetes mellitus. *JAMA*, 286, 327-334.

[208] Tausk, F., Elenkov, I., Moynihan, J. (2008) Psychoneuroimmunology. Dermatol. Ther, 21:22-31.

[209] Dentino. A,N,, Pieper. C,F,, Rao. M,K,, Currie MS, Harris T, Blazer DG, Cohen HJ. (1999) Association of interleukin-6 and other biologic variables with depression in older people living in the community. *J. Am. Geriatr Soc*, 47, 6-11.

[210] Dhabhar, F.S. (2003) Stress, leukocyte trafficking, and the augmentation of skin immune function. *Ann. N. Y. Acad. Sci*, 992, 205-217.

In: Immunology in Clinic Practice
Editor: Cagatay Oktenli, pp. 115-136

ISBN 978-1-60876-644-4


*Chapter 7*

# CURRENT PERSPECTIVES ON IMMUNOLOGY AND ENDOCRINOLOGY

***Çağatay Öktenli and Serkan Çelik***
Division of Internal Medicine,
GATA Haydarpasa Training Hospital, Istanbul, Turkey

## ABSTRACT

Sex steroids and their metabolites and receptors are all involved in immunoregulation, suggesting sex steroids influence the development and function of the immune system cells. Proinflammatory cytokines are potent activators of the hypothalamic-pituitary-adrenal axis primarily at the level of the brain and/or pituitary gland. Increased evidence has provided that the immune system modifies bone functions through a complex intreaction involving dendritic cells, T and B cells, cytokines, and cell-signaling pathways, which are in turn further modified by hormones such as leptin, vitamin D, parathyroid hormone, and testosterone.

**Keywords:** immune-neuro–endocrine; hypothalamic-pituitary-adrenal axis; hypothalamic–pituitary–thyroid and gonadal axes; obesity; bone metabolism

## INTRODUCTION

Accumulating evidence demonstrates that the immune and neuroendocrine systems communicate bidirectionally [1]. In this way, the immune-neuro–endocrine interface is mediated by cytokines and they are produced within the hypothalamic-pituitary-adrenal axis itself [2]. Cytokines may also exert local regulatory actions on hormone release, pituitary-cell development and feedback control of the hypothalamic-pituitary-adrenal axis [1,3]. These cytokines are also to suppress growth hormone release, and the hypothalamic–pituitary–thyroid and gonadal axes [1].

## The Relation between Immune System and Hypothalamic-pituitary-adrenal Axis

Proinflammatory cytokines are potent activators of the hypothalamic-pituitary-adrenal axis primarily at the level of the brain and/or pituitary gland [4,5]. In addition, cytokines may cause a change in the pain responses, behavior and mood [6-8]. Furthermore, in recent studies [9-11], (1) cytokines induce ACTH release, (2) local synthesis of these cytokines is regulated by the lipopolysaccharide (LPS) receptors on folliculostellate cells, and the synthesis is augmented by stimuli such as infection and inflammation.

In the adrenal gland, cytokines enhance the rise in circulating glucocorticoids, while a concomitant acute reduction in circulating corticosteroid-binding globulin facilitates the delivery of the steroids to the tissues [12,13]. It has been reported that exposure to endotoxin produces a significant increase in adrenal IL-6 and IL-1β expression [14]. Classically, glucocorticoids exert potent modulatory effects on immunity through the glucocorticoid receptor localized in the cytoplasm and complexed to heat-shock proteins [15]. They suppress the inflammatory response genes and the Toll receptor signaling [7]. Glucocorticoids stimulate the production of various antiinflammatory cytokines and also inhibit the production of proinflammatory cytokines and metalloproteinases [16]. Interestingly, recent evidence demonstrates that glucocorticoid receptor represses inflammatory responses genes [17]. On the other hand, it has been reported that the feedback actions of the glucocorticoids are less effective in chronic immune activation, possibly because of the expression of a dominant negative isoform of the glucocorticoids [18]. Additionally, leptin, IL-4, IL-10, melanocyte-stimulating hormone and transforming growth factor β (TGF- β), may modulate the hypothalamic-pituitary-adrenal response to pro-inflammatory cytokines [12]. Macrophage migration inhibitory factor is also produced by the pituitary corticotrophs and it suppress the inhibitory effects of glucocorticoids [19,20].

## Sex Steroids and Immune System

Sex steroids and their metabolites and receptors are all involved in immunoregulation, suggesting sex steroids influence the development and function of the immune system cells [16,21,22]. Estrogens are enhancers at least of the humoral immunity and androgens and progesterone are natural immune-suppressors [23,24]. Thus, females have a higher immunoglobulin (Ig) levels and stronger immune responses following immunization or infection than males [25]. This is also evident in their increased susceptibility to autoimmune diseases [25,26]. In addition, lymphoid organs and peripheral immune cells express gonadotropin releasing hormone and their receptors [27]. It has been reported that gonadotropin releasing hormone is also involved in thymus maturation and has a potent immune-stimulating action increasing the levels of some cytokines (IFN-γ, IL-2), and T helper (Th) cells [22].

## Cellular Immunity

### *T Cells*

Accumulating evidence demonstrates that sex hormones play an important role in the regulation of the T cells. Normally, total T cell count in males is similar to females [28,29]. However, since testosterone may increase apoptosis in T cells [30], the percentage of T cells within the total T cell population in males is lower than females [29]. Estrogen can cause a reduction in the number of immature thymic lymphocytes and in the mass of thymic stromal tissue [22,31]. Estrogen can alter the comparative subsets of mature T cells to one favoring the Th-cell phenotype [22]. Estrogen can also activate an extra-thymic pathway of autoreactive T cell differentiation [22]. Prolactin is a T cell mitogen and the action of prolactin is mediated by prolactin receptor/Janus activating kinase (JAK)/Stat/IRF-1 signaling pathway [32,33]. Androgens influence the size and composition of the thymus [51]. They have a direct or indirect effect on enhance suppressor effect increasing CD4- CD8+ cells [51]. In mice models, the administration of testosterone causes a shift in the proportion of T cells to one favoring the T-suppressor-cell phenotype [34].

Classically, one of the main functions of Th cells is the production of cytokines [35]. IFN-γ is one of the cytokines playing an important role in specific immune responses. In previous studies, effects of sex hormones on lymphocyte IFN-γ production was not reported [36,37]. But, recent studies demonstrated that high levels of estrogen and prolactin can increase IFN-γ and IL-2 by Th1 lymphocytes activation [6,22,38]. IL-2 is another major cytokine responsible for T cell activation and proliferation [35]. It has been reported that, as compared to female lymphocytes, IL-2 production is to be similar [36] or decreased in stimulated male lymphocytes [29]. IL-4 is released predominantly by Th2 cells and it is an important growth promoting factor for Th2 cells [35]. In contrast to other researcher [36], Faas et al. reported that the production of IL-4 in ovarian cycle is significantly increased in Th cells in the luteal phase as compared with the follicular phase [39]. On the other hand, it has been reported that IL-2 and IL-4 reduced prolactin mRNA levels in T lymphocytes [40].

### *Monocytes*

It is well known that monocytes are able to ingest and kill pathogens by the process of phagocytosis [35]. It has been proposed that estrogen and progesterone can decrease monocyte numbers [41]. This may be due to sex hormones inducing apoptosis and mitotic arrest in monocytes [41]. Estrogen also inhibits the Th1 cytokine production, and stimulates the Th2 cytokine production [28,42,43]. However, other authors reported that 17β-estradiol (17β-$E_2$) and progesterone do not influence the production of cytokine in women [44]. TNF-α is one of the cytokine secreted by activated macrophages and monocytes. Interestingly, physiologic concentrations of 17β-$E_2$ have been suggested to inhibit TNF-α [45]. Moreover, it has been reported that endotoxin-stimulated monocytes produce more TNF-α in males than females [29]. Although testosterone specifically targets CD8+CD4+ thymocytes for apoptosis via upgrading TNF-α production [46], other researchers reported that there is no effect of testosterone upon monocyte TNF-α production [37]. Similarly, differences in IL-1β synthesis at different hormonal stages were reported [35]. In this way, percentage IL-1β producing in stimulated monocytes was higher in males than females [29] and 17β-$E_2$ and/or progesterone exert monocyte IL-1β production [47]. In addition, it has been also suggested that incubation of whole blood with physiological concentrations of testosterone increased monocyte IL-1ß production [37]. However, in experimental studies, there is no effect of both sex hormones on endotoxin-stimulated monocytes IL-1β production [19]. IL-6 is the other cytokine produced by monocytes and macrophages [35]. It has been suggested that stimulated IL-6 production was either decreased [48] or not affected [49] by the estrogenic compound in hormone replasman therapy. Estrogen-mediated down-regulation of IL-6 expression may also involve inhibitory effects on NF-κB pathways [50]. IL-12 is another important cytokine that links the non-specific to the specific immune system [35]. *In vitro*, a decreasing effect of 17β-$E_2$ on IL-12 production was reported, whereas progesterone did not affect the production of this cytokine [51]. It has been suggested that physiological levels of testosterone can enhance IL-12 production by LPS-stimulated monocytes [37]. On the other hand, prolactin triggers release of IL-12 [52].

### *Dendritic Cells*

It has been demonstrated that in the presence of progesteron and estradiol can cause alterations of the immunomodulatory functions of the monocyte-derived dendritic cells [53]. In experimental studies, it has been demonstrated that estrogen augments the number of potent antigen-presenting cells by promoting the differentiation of dendritic cells [54]. Conversely, *in vitro* estrogen exposure reduces the capacity of mature dendritic cells [43]. On the other hand, prolactin may participate in dendritic cell maturation [55]. It has been reported that prolactin upregulate GM-CSF receptors, leading to synergistically induced maturation of immature dendritic cells [26]. Furthermore, prolonged incubation of dendritic cells with prolactin induces antigen-presenting activity [56].

### *Neutrophils*

There are little information about the effects of sex hormones on neutrophil functions [35]. Neutrophil free radical production has been reported to be increased [57], decreased [58] or not affected [59] by estrogen or progesterone incubations *in vitro*.

### *Natural Killer (NK) Cells*

Classically, NK cells, in the absence of prior immunization, are capable of killing tumour or virus-infected cells and are able to lyse these target cells by direct contact [35]. Although there is no difference could be demonstrated in NK cell count between males and females [28], it has been demonstrated that estrogen can decrease NK cell counts [47]. Furthermore, NK cell activity was higher in post-menopausal women and in males than young females, suggesting a suppression of NK cell activity by progesterone or 17ß-$E_2$ [60].

## Humoral Immunity

### *B Cells*

The effects of estrogens on B cell development were suggested in previous studies [26,61,62]. In mice, estrogens can increase progenitor B cells by protecting the bone marrow progenitor cells from apoptosis [61,62]. However, estrogen effects are not only limited to B cell development in the bone marrow, but also extend to peripheral lymphoid organs [26]. In this context, B cell numbers in the blood, lymph nodes and spleen are under estrogen control [63]. Estrogen may also influence B lymphocyte subsets and peripheral B cell development [35,64]. Although it has been suggested that B1 subsets remained stable after menopause, the B2 subset decreased after menopause [65]. On the other hand, prolactin plays a role in the regulation of the B lymphocyte pool size [26]. Experimental studies show that prolactin can also impact B cell maturation in peripheral lymphoid organs [66] and can promote B cell survival [67].

The effects of estrogen on B lymphopoiesis have not yet been completely elucidated [26]. On the one hand, it was proposed that estrogen regulates B lymphopoiesis only indirectly, through its effect on stromal cells [68]. However, other studies have shown that estrogen directly affects early pro-B cells [69]. Possibly, this estrogen effect is mediated by estrogen receptor (ER)α and Erβ. In this way, both receptors are expressed on B cell progenitors of mice [26]. On the other hand, estrogen decreases IgM-mediated apoptosis of transitional B cells, thereby interfering with an important mechanism for negative selection of autoreactive B cells [70]. Therefore, these estrogen effects on B cell development may decrease negative selection in naïve immature B cells [61]. This may be related with higher incidence of autoimmune diseases in women [35].

The production of antibodies is the main functions of B cells [35]. Interestingly, women have higher serum levels of total IgG and IgM than men [28]. Patients with Klinefelter syndrome have higher immunoglobulin levels, and with androgen administration, antibody levels diminish and approximate quantities seen in healthy male subjects [71]. Resembling changes were reported in male patients with idiopathic hypogonadotrophic hypogonadism before and after gonadotroping treatment; testosterone normalisation was associated with a decrease in immunoglobulin levels [72].

## Bone Metabolism and Immune System

Increased evidence has provided that the immune system modifies bone functions through a complex intreaction involving T and B cells, dendritic cells, cytokines, and cell-signaling pathways, which are in turn further modified by circulating hormones such as vitamin D, parathyroid hormone, testosterone, and leptin [73]. It has been well known that infection, inflammation, and autoimmune disorders are associated with systemic and local bone loss [74].

T cells may regulate osteoclast and osteoblast formation, lifespan, and activity [75-79]. Osteoclasts arise by cytokine-driven proliferation and differentiation of hematopoietic precursors [80]. It has been recently suggested that the cytokines required for osteoclast formation are receptor activator of nuclear factor κB ligand (RANKL) and macrophage colony-stimulating factor (M-CSF) [74]. Particularly, the TNF-family molecule RANKL and its receptor RANK are key regulators of bone remodelling [81]. They are essential for the development and activation of osteoclasts [81]. In this manner, RANKL binds to the transmembrane receptor RANK, which is expressed on the surface of osteoclasts and osteoclast precursors [74]. In addition, RANKL binds to osteoprotogerin, known as osteoclastogenesis inhibitory factor [74]. Osteoprotogerin by sequestering RANKL and preventing its binding to RANK [80,82]. On the other hand, M-CSF induces the proliferation of early osteoclast precursors and the differentiation of more mature osteoclasts [74].

TNF, another important cytokine, enhances osteoclast formation by upregulating the stromal cell production of RANKL and M-CSF [83]. It has been reported that the ability of TNF to increase the osteoclastogenic activity of RANKL is due to synergistic interactions at the level of NFκB and activator protein-1 signaling [83]. Furthermore, TNF inhibits osteoblastogenesis, whereas it stimulates osteoclast activity [84]. It has been also reported that IL-1 mediates the osteclastogenic effect of TNF [85]. Interestingly, IFN-γ, a potent inhibitor of osteoclastogenesis *in vitro,* was previously accepted as an anti-osteoclastogenic cytokine [71]. IFN-γ can prevent uncontrolled bone loss during inflammatory T cell responses [86] and can inhibit RANKL induced osteoclast differentiation [87]. Senescent T cells show an impaired IFN-γ production and this may be related increasing incidence of osteoporosis during senescence [88]. On the other hand, elevated IL-6 levels [89] and the presence of high expression IL-6 alleles [90] enhance the risk of osteoporosis [91]. In addition, parathyroid hormone stimulates production of IL-6 [92]. IL-4 is another anti-osteoclastogenic cytokine and it can act through STAT6-dependent inhibition of NFκB signaling [93]. Another cytokine relevant for osteoclast formation is IL-7 [94]. It has been reported that IL-12 inhibits osteoclast formation *in vitro* [95]. On the other hand, TGF-β is another factor that plays a key, complex, and controversial role in osteoclastogenesis [96].

Although cytokines participate in inflammatory events throughout the body, in bone, hormonal status and cytokine function are closely related [77-79]. Consequently, local effects of estrogens and androgens on bone metabolism may be direct or indirect, with the indirect effects mediated principally via cytokines [97].

## Obesity and Immune Functions

Accumulating evidence have suggested a link between immunity and metabolism [98-100]. In this manner, immune system signals may directly influence the metabolic axis. Reciprocally, energy balance and metabolism of the body may potentially exert potent effects on immune function and trafficking [100]. In both humans and obese rodents, it has been reported that excess adiposity can cause impaired immune functions [98]. On the other hand, adipose lineage cells show macrophage properties such as microbicidal and phagocytic activities [101,102]. In a more recent report, it has been suggested that obesity constricts T-cell diversity by accelerating thymic aging [103]. Another source of evidence comes from adipose tissue-secreted proteins such as leptin, adiponectin, resistin, IL-1, TNF-α, IL-6, IL-8, IFN-γ, TGF-β, chemokines, adipsin and acylation stimulating protein [104]. These proteins are called adipokines.

Since its cloning in 1994, the role of leptin, which well known adipokine released by adipose tissue, in regulating immune and inflammatory response has become increasingly evident [105-106]. Previous studies have suggested that several immune cells express leptin receptors [105]. Leptin has also certain structural similarities to cytokines such as IL-6, GM-CSF or IL-12 [107]. Leptin modulates the functions and proleferation of naïve T cells, whereas only promotes the secretion of Th1 cytokines [107-110]. In this way, leptin directly stimulate expression and release of IL-1, IL-6, IFN-γ, and TNF-α [111,112]. Moreover, leptin acts as an acute-phase reactant during inflammation [113]. It has been proposed that leptin has a selective thymo-stimulatory role in settings of leptin deficiency [114,115]. Leptin-deficient ob/ob mice also show impaired phagocytosis of *Klebsiella pneumoniae* [116]. On the other hand, addition of leptin to a mixed lymphocyte reaction induces a dose-dependent increase in CD4 T cell proliferation [117]. In neutrophils, leptin leads to an increase neutrophil chemotaxis and the release of reactive oxygen species [107,118,119]. Furthermore, leptin can regulate NK cells by affecting proliferation, differentiation, activation and cytotoxicity [120]. Consequently, recent evidence suggests a role for leptin in the pathogenesis of some autoimmune diseases [121] and administration of leptin triggers the onset and accelerates the progression of autoimmune diseases [122].

Adiponectin is a second well known adipocytokine released by fat cells and it has several beneficial and protective effects on metabolism [115]. Adiponectin induces IL-10 and IL-1RA in monocytes, macrophages, and dendritic cells [123]. Conversely, adiponectin significantly blocks proinflammatory cytokines production and decreases phagocytotic capacity of macrophages [123,124]. Adiponectin is also able to inhibit Toll-receptor activation and its consequences [125]. Adiponectin suppresses the IL-2-enhanced cytotoxic activity of NK cells [126]. Adiponectin inhibits B lymphopoiesis [127].

Resistin is a 114 amino-acid peptide and its effects on the immune system are relatively poorly investigated [115]. It has been reported that resistin mRNA has been observed in peripheral blood mononuclear cells and was increased by pre-treatment with cytokines [128]. Interestingly, resistin itself leads to increased release of TNF-α and IL-12 [129]. Furthermore, it has been also suggested that resistin were able to activate these cytokines suggesting that the inflammatory action of resistin is independent of its conformation [129].

Visfatin, originally identified as a pre-B-cell colony-enhancing factor, has recently been identified as an adipocytokine secreted by adipocytes in visceral fat [130,131]. It has been reported that visfatin activates leukocytes and induces cytokine production [132]. In addition, visfatin induces the production of IL-1, IL-6 and TNF-α in CD14+ monocytes. Moreover, visfatin upregulates surface expression of costimulatory molecules (CD40, CD54, and CD80). Furthermore, it has been reported that visfatin stimulates monocytes and increases capacity to induce alloproliferative responses on lymphocytes [132].

Adipsin is secreted in adipose tissue. It has complement factor D activity and catalyzes the first activation step in the alternative pathway of complement [133]. Moreover, adipocytes produce factor D and C3 of the complement cascade. These observations suggest a link between adipsin and the complement alternative pathway with obesity.

Ghrelin functions as a positive regulator of the somatotropic axis and a peripheral signal of negative energy balance [100]. Ghrelin mRNA is expressed in the spleen, thymus, lymph nodes, and peripheral T cells, monocytes and dendritic cells [100,134]. Therefore, ghrelin also exerts multiple regulatory effects on immune systems [100]. In this way, it has been reported that ghrelin exerts potent inhibitory effects on the proinflammatory cytokines [111]. Xia et al. also demonstrated that ghrelin inhibits proliferation of anti-CD3 activated murine T cells and non-specifically inhibits both Th1 and Th2 cytokines [135].

It is well know that IL-1 inhibit fatty acid synthesis and adipocyte differentiation [136]. Interestingly, IL-1 also promotes the release of neuropeptides such as the melanocortins, corticotropin-releasing hormone, and α-melanocyte-stimulating hormone [136]. IL-1Ra-deficient mice are lean and resistant to high-fat-diet-induced obesity [136]. Conversely, IL-1-Ra levels correlate with insulin resistance [137].

IL-6 is another important cytokine associated with obesity [138]. IL-6 regulates B-cell development, antibody production and adipocyte or metabolic function. Moreover, the IL-6 receptor (IL-6R) is homologous to the leptin receptor. IL-6 and IL-6R are expressed by adipocytes [139]. IL-6 secretion are 2 to 3 times greater in visceral relative to subcutaneous adipose tissue [139,140]. Adipose tissue IL-6 expression and circulating IL-6 concentrations are positively correlated with obesity [103]. It has been suggested that genetic polymorphisms of the IL-6 locus have been linked to obesity [138]. On the other hand, mice with a targeted deletion of IL-6 develop mature-onset obesity and associated metabolic abnormalities [141].

TNF-α has been implicated in the pathogenesis of obesity and insulin resistance [142,143]. TNF-α is expressed by adipocytes [99]. Moreover, TNF-α expression is greater in subcutaneous compared with visceral adipose tissue [139,140]. Adipocytes also express both types of TNF-α receptors and soluble forms [143]. Adipose tissue expression of TNF-α is increased in obese rodents and humans and is positively correlated with adiposity [142,143]. It has also been reported that patients with insulin resistance have increased levels of TNF-α and that TNF-α-deficient mice are protected from insulin resistance [144]. In this manner, release of soluble TNF receptors can neutralize unbound circulating TNF-α and inhibit both the subsequent development of TNF-α-induced insulin resistance and adipogenesis [145]. On the other hand, TNF-α influences gene expression in adipose tissue [146]. TNF-α suppresses genes for transcription factors involved in adipogenesis and lipogenesis [146]. TNF-α suppresses expression of genes involved in glucose uptake and metabolism and fatty acid oxidation [146]. It also increases expression of genes involved in de novo synthesis of cholesterol and fatty acids in liver [146].

IFN-γ is another cytokine that might play a central role during hypermetabolic and anorectic responses associated with inflammation. It has been reported that IFN-γ-receptor-deficient mice are protected from lipopolysaccharide-induced anorexia [147].

MCP-1, a chemokine, is expressed and secreted by adipose tissue [148]. Both adipose tissue expression of MCP-1 and circulating MCP-1 levels are increased in rodent obesity, suggesting that MCP-1-mediated macrophage infiltration of adipose tissue may contribute to the metabolic abnormalities associated with obesity [149,150]. MCP-1 also inhibits adipocyte growth and differentiation by decreasing the expression of a number of adipogenic genes [150,151]. In rodent obesity, increased circulating MCP-1 is associated with increased circulating monocytes [149].

## Immune System and Regulation of Hypothalamus-Pituitary-Thyroid Axis

Classically, the primary function of the hypothalamus-pituitary-thyroid axis is to regulate thyroid hormone synthesis and production. Thyrotropin-releasing hormone serves as an inductive signal for the release of thyrotropin (TSH) from the anterior pituitary. Finally, TSH induces the release of thyroxine (T4) and triiodothyronine (T3). In this manner, initial studies suggested that TSH produced by immune system cells like leukocytes and dendritic cells [152-155]. TSH could exert an effect on cells of the body: one being a direct effect of TSH on cells of the immune system, the other being an indirect effect mediated by thyroid hormone [152]. TSH may act as a cytokine-like regulatory molecule within the immune system [152].

Bagriacik et al. demonstrated the expression of thyroid stimulating hormone receptor (TSH-R) on lymphoid and myeloid cells [156]. TSH also could act indirectly on the immune system by altering thyroid T3 and T4 release. Thus, they affect the functional or developmental activity of cells in the bone marrow and in secondary lymphoid tissues [152].

Euthyroid sick syndrome is a hypothyroidic condition that occurs in the absence of overt thyroid disease [152,157]. In experimental models for euthyroid sick syndrome, two mechanisms have been suggested for suppressed TSH levels [152]. First, infusion of rats with the proinflammatory cytokines has been shown to lower serum TSH levels [152]. Second, research has demonstrated that T4 is converted to T3 in tanycytes of the third ventricle near the hypothalamic median eminence, thereby causing a surge in T3 locally [158].

## Autoimmune Thyroid Diseases

Recent researches have focused on the autoantigens in autoimmune thyroid disease (AITD) [159-165]. Graves' disease is an organ-specific autoimmune disease of the thyroid gland [160]. Immunological features of Graves' disease include lymphocytic infiltration of the thyroid gland and circulating autoantibodies against thyroglobulin, thyroid peroxidase and the TSH-R [160,161]. A form of autoimmune hypothyroidism, Hashimoto's thyroiditis, was first described in 1912 by Hashimoto and is now recognised as the major form of chronic autoimmune thyroiditis [160].

Conceptually, cytokine patterns in both Graves' disease and autoimmune hypothyroidism reveal both a Th1 and Th2 response. In a murine model, immune deviation towards Th2 was accompanied by a decrease, while Th1 responses to TSH-R were critical for disease induction [164]. Moreover, IFN-γ are not associated with the development of AITD despite the key role of this cytokine in Th1 pattern [166]. On the other hand, some chemokines have been reported to be overexpressed in AITD patients with thyroid germinal centres [167].

The involvement of the thyroid follicular cells is a key feature of AITD [159]. In this way, the induction of MHC class II expression on thyroid follicular cells is critically dependent on IFN-γ [159]. In response to IL-1 and TNF-α or chemokines, thyroid follicular cells themselves secrete an increasingly well identified array of cytokines [167,168].

The mechanisms by which AITD develop are unclear, although it is likely that AITD occur in genetically susceptible individuals exposed to a permissive environment [160]. The first AITD susceptibility gene locus identified was the human leukocyte antigen DR (HLA-DR) gene locus and on this basis Graves' disease was assumed to be a straightforward HLA-class II-restricted autoantibody response to the TSH-R [169]. In the past, associations between Graves' disease and HLA-DR3 and specifically the DRB1*0304-DQB1*02-DQA1*0501 haplotype have been reported [160,170]. Recent evidence provided a primary association of HLA class I genes and Graves' disease, which is stronger than that observed with class II genes and pointing to a primary role for class I-mediated responses in Graves' disease [171]. The CTLA-4 gene has been investigated as a candidate for the development of Graves' disease because of its role in down-regulating the immune system [160]. Takara et al. [172] replicated A to G polymorphism findings in Japanese patients with younger-onset type 1 diabetes and autoimmune thyroid disease. Other researchers have also suggested the CTLA-4 A/G polymorphism to be linked to thyroid autoantibody production [173]. The interleukin-1 receptor antagonist (IL-1ra) gene and a number of other susceptibility genes have also been investigated as a candidate for Graves' disease [160]. A C to T polymorphism at –590 in the promoter region of the interleukin-4 (IL-4) gene was reported to confer protection to Graves' disease [174]. However, information from a much larger study has raised serious questions of these findings [175]. Finally, Jacobson and Tomer [176] have divided the identified AITD susceptibility genes into two groups: (1) immune-modulating genes (HLA-DR, CD40, CTLA-4, and PTPN22 genes) and (2) thyroid-specific genes (thyroglobulin and TSH-R genes).

Consequently, Hashimoto's thyroiditis patients exhibited a reduced percentage of NK and CD25+-bearing cells, thus indicating the presence of a certain degree of peripheral immune deficiency [177]. In addition, an increased percentage of the naive (CD25+ CD45RA+) subpopulation of Th and of CD8+ lymphocytes in both Graves' disease and Hashimoto's thyroiditis patients was demonstrated compared to healthy volunteers [177]. Moreover, it has been suggested that hypothyroid experimental conditions lead to spleen and lymph node involution and restoration of thyroid function improved both humoral and cell-mediated immune responses [178,179].

## Conclusion

GnRH and sex steroids seem to play an important role as modulators of the autoimmune disease onset/perpetuation. The accumulating data suggest that obesity can be regarded as an inflammatory disease. The causative factors of this inflammation process are not entirely understood, but adipose tissue seems to play an important role in the relationship between obesity and chronic inflammation. A better understanding of the mechanisms of obesity induced inflammatory response might lead to identifying novel therapeutic targets to prevent obesity-related complications.

## References

[1] Haddad, J.J., Saade, N.E., Safieh-Garabedian, B. (2002) Cytokines and neuro-immune-endocrine interactions: a role for the hypothalamic-pituitary-adrenal revolving axis. *J. Neuroimmunol*, 133, 1-19.

[2] Chesnokova, V., Melmed, S., (2002), Minireview: Neuro-immuno-endocrine modulation of the hypothalamic-pituitary-adrenal (HPA) axis by gp130 signaling molecules. *Endocrinology*, 143, 1571–4.

[3] Raison, C..L, Borisov, A.S., Majer, M., Drake, D.F., Pagnoni, G., Woolwine, B.J., Vogt, G.J., Massung, B., Miller, A.H. (2009) Activation of central nervous system inflammatory pathways by interferon-alpha: relationship to monoamines and depression. *Biol. Psychiatry*, 65, 296-303.

[4] Liege, S., Moze, E., Kelley, K.W., Parnet, P., Neveu, P.J. (2000) Activation of the hypothalamic-pituitary-adrenal axis in IL-1 beta-converting enzyme-deficient mice. *Neuroimmunomodulation*, 7, 189–94.

[5] Elenkov, I.J., Wilder, R.L., Chrousos, G.P., Vizi E.S. (2000) The sympathetic nerve--an integrative interface between two supersystems: the brain and the immune system. *Pharmacol. Rev*, 52, 595–638.

[6] Eskandari, F., Webster, J.I., Sternberg, E.M. (2003) Neural immune pathways and their connection to inflammatory diseases. *Arthritis Res. Ther*, 5, 251–265.

[7] Turrin, N.P., Rivest, S. (2004) Unraveling the molecular details involved in the intimate link between the immune and neuroendocrine systems. *Exp. Biol. Med*, 229, 996–1006.

[8] Chida, D., Imaki, T., Suda, T., Iwakura, Y. (2005) Involvement of corticotropin-releasing hormone- and interleukin (IL)-6-dependent proopiomelanocortin induction in the anterior pituitary during hypothalamic-pituitary-adrenal axis activation by IL-1alpha. *Endocrinology*, 146, 5496–502.

[9] Arzt, E. (2001) gp130 cytokine signaling in the pituitary gland: a paradigm for cytokine-neuro-endocrine pathways. *J. Clin. Invest*, 108, 1729–33.

[10] Gloddek, J., Lohrer, P., Stalla, J., Arzt, E., Stalla, G.K., Renner, U. (2001) The intrapituitary stimulatory effect of lipopolysaccharide on ACTH secretion is mediated by paracrine-acting IL-6. *Exp. Clin. Endocrinol. Diabetes*, 109, 410–415.

[11] Chesnokova, V., Melmed, S. (2000) Leukemia inhibitory factor mediates the hypothalamic pituitary adrenal axis response to inflammation. *Endocrinology*, 141, 4032–4040.

[12] John, C.D., Buckingham, J.C. (2003) Cytokines: regulation of the hypothalamo-pituitary-adrenocortical axis. *Curr. Opin. Pharmacol*, 3, 78-84.

[13] Beishuizen, A., Thijs, L.G., Vermes, I. (2001) Patterns of corticosteroid-binding globulin and the free cortisol index during septic shock and multitrauma. *Intensive Care Med*, 27, 1584–1591.

[14] Cover, P.O., Slater, D., Buckingham, J.C. (2001) Expression of cyclooxygenase enzymes in rat hypothalamo-pituitary-adrenal axis: effects of endotoxin and glucocorticoids. *Endocrine*, 16, 123–131.

[15] Yeager, M.P., Guyre, P.M., Munck, A.U. (2004) Glucocorticoid regulation of the inflammatory response to injury. *Acta Anaesthesiol. Scand*, 48, 799-813.

[16] Jara, L.J., Navarro, C., Medina, G., Vera-Lastra, O., Blanco, F. (2006) Immune-neuroendocrine interactions and autoimmune diseases. *Clin. Dev. Immun*, 13, 109-123.

[17] Ogawa, S., Lozach, J., Benner, C., Pascual, G., Tangirala, R.K., Westin, S., Hoffmann, A., Subramaniam, S., David, M., Rosenfeld, M.G., Glass, C.K. (2005) Molecular determinants of crosstalk between nuclear receptors and toll-like receptors. *Cell*, 122, 707-721.

[18] Webster, J.C., Oakley, R.H., Jewell, C.M., Cidlowski, J.A. (2001) Proinflammatory cytokines regulate human glucocorticoid receptor gene expression and lead to the accumulation of the dominant negative beta isoform: a mechanism for the generation of glucocorticoid resistance. *Proc. Natl. Acad. Sci. USA*, 98, 6865–6870.

[19] Daun, J.M., and Cannon, J.G. (2000) Macrophage migration inhibitory factor antagonizes hydrocortisone-induced increases in cytosolic IkappaBalpha. *Am. J. Physiol. Regul. Integr. Comp. Physiol*, 279, R1043–1049.

[20] Isidori, A.M., Kaltsas, G.A., Korbonits, M., Pyle, M., Gueorguiev, M., Meinhardt, A., Metz, C., Petrovsky, N., Popovic, V., Bucala, R., et al. (2002) Response of serum macrophage migration inhibitory factor levels to stimulation or suppression of the

hypothalamo-pituitary-adrenal axis in normal subjects and patients with Cushing's disease. *J. Clin. Endocrinol. Metab*, 87, 1834–1840.

[21] Ackerman, L.S. (2006) Sex hormones and the genesis of autoimmunity. *Arch Dermatol*, 142, 371-376.

[22] Tanriverdi, F., Silveira, L.F.G., MacColl, G.S., Bouloux, P.M.G. (2003) Sex hormones and the genesis of autoimmunity. *J. Endocrinol*, 176, 293.

[23] Cutolo, M., Villaggio, B., Craviotto, C., Pizzorni, C., Seriolo, B., Sulli, A. (2002) Sex hormones and rheumatoid arthritis. *Autoimmun. Rev*, 1, 284-289.

[24] Cutolo, M., and Wilder, R. (2000) Different roles for androgens and estrogens in the susceptibility to autoimmune rheumatic diseases. *Rheum. Dis. Clin. North Am*, 26, 825-839.

[25] Verthelyi, D. (2001) Sex hormones as immunomodulators in health and disease. *Int. Immunopharmacol*, 1, 983-993.

[26] Peeva, E., Zouali, M. (2005) Spotlight on the role of hormonal factors in the emergence of autoreactive B-lymphocytes. *Immunol. Lett*, 101, 123-143.

[27] Silveira, L.F., Stewart, P.M., Thomas, M., Clark, D.A., Bouloux, P.M., MacColl, G.S. (2002) Novel homozygous splice acceptor site GnRH receptor (GnRHR) mutation: human GnRHR "knockout". *J. Clin. Endocrinol. Metab*, 87, 2973-2977.

[28] Giltay, E.J., Fonk, J.C., von Blomberg, B.M., Drexhage, H.A., Schalkwijk, C., Gooren, L.J. (2000) In vivo effects of sex steroids on lymphocyte responsiveness and immunoglobulin levels in humans. *J. Clin. Endocrinol. Metab*, 85, 1648-1657.

[29] Bouman, A., Schipper, M., Heineman, M.J., Faas, M.M. (2004) Gender difference in the non-specific and specific immune response in humans. *Am. J. Reprod. Immunol*, 52, 19-26.

[30] McMurray, R.W., Suwannaroj, S., Ndebele, K., Jenkins, J.K. (2001) Differential effects of sex steroids on T and B cells: modulation of cell cycle phase distribution, apoptosis and bcl-2 protein levels. *Pathobiology*, 69, 44-58.

[31] Maret, A., Coudert, J.D., Garidou, L., Foucras, G., Gourdy, P., Krust, A., Dupont, S., Chambon, P., Druet, P., Bayard, F., Guéry, J.C. (2003) Estradiol enhances primary antigen-specific CD4 T cell responses and Th1 development in vivo. Essential role of estrogen receptor alpha expression in hematopoietic cells. *Eur. J. Immunol*, 33, 512-521.

[32] Vera-Lastra, O., Jara, L.J., Espinoza, L.R. (2002) Prolactin and autoimmunity. *Autoimmun. Rev*, 1, 360–364.

[33] Yu-Lee, L.Y. (2002) Prolactin modulation of immune and inflammatory responses. *Recent Prog. Horm. Res*, 57, 435–455.

[34] De León-Nava, M.A., Nava, K., Soldevila, G., López-Griego, L., Chávez-Ríos, J.R., Vargas-Villavicencio, J.A., Morales-Montor, J. (2009) Immune sexual dimorphism: effect of gonadal steroids on the expression of cytokines, sex steroid receptors, and lymphocyte proliferation. *J. Steroid Biochem. Mol. Biol*, 113, 57-64.

[35] Bouman, A., Heineman, M.J., Faas M.M. (2005) Sex hormones and the immune response in humans. *Hum. Reprod. Update*, 4, 411-423.

[36] Giron-Gonzalez, J.A., Moral, F.J., Elvira, J., Garcia-Gil, D., Guerrero, F., Gavilan, I. Escobar, L. (2000) Consistent production of a higher TH1:TH2 cytokine ratio by stimulated T cells in men compared with women. *Eur. J. Endocrinol*, 143, 31-36.

[37] Posma, E., Moes, H., Heineman, M.J. Faas, M. (2004) The effect of testosterone on cytokine production in the specific and non-specific immune response. *Am. J. Reprod. Immunol*, 52, 237-243.

[38] Lang, T.J. (2004) Estrogen as an immunomodulator. *Clin. Immunol*, 113, 224–230.

[39] Faas, M., Bouman, A., Moes, H., Heineman, M.J., de Leij, L., Schuiling, G. (2000) The immune response during the luteal phase of the ovarian cycle: a Th2-type response? *Fertil Steril*, 74, 1008-1013.

[40] Gerlo, S., Verdood, P., Hooghe-Peters, E.L., Kooijman, R. (2005) Modulation of prolactin expression in human T lymphocytes by cytokines. *J. Neuroimmunol*, 162, 190–193.

[41] Thongngarm, T., Jenkins, J.K., Ndebele, K., McMurray, R.W. (2003) Estrogen and progesterone modulate monocyte cell cycle progression and apoptosis. *Am. J. Reprod. Immunol*, 49, 129-138.

[42] Salem, M. (2004) Estrogen, a double-edged sword: modulation of TH1- and TH2-mediated inflammations by differential regulation of TH1/TH2 cytokine production. *Curr. Drug Targets Inflamm. Allergy*, 3, 97-104.

[43] Liu, H., Buenafe, A.C., Matejuk, A., Ito, A., Zamora, A., Dwyer J., et al. (2002) Estrogen inhibition of EAE involves effects on dendritic cell function. *J. Neurosci. Res*, 70, 238-248.

[44] Bouman, A., Schipper, M., Heineman, M.J., Faas, M. (2004) 17beta-estradiol and progesterone do not influence the production of cytokines from lipopolysaccharide-stimulated monocytes in humans. *Fertil Steril*, 82, 1212-1219.

[45] Lambert, K.C., Curran, E.M., Judy, B.M., Lubahn D.B., Estes, D.M. (2004) Estrogen receptor-alpha deficiency promotes increased TNF-alpha secretion and bacterial killing by murine macrophages in response to microbial stimuli in vitro. *J. Leukoc. Biol*, 75, 1166-1172.

[46] Guevara Patino, J.A., Marino, M.W., Ivanov, V.N., Nikolich-Zugich, J. (2000) Sex steroids induce apoptosis of CD8+CD4+ double-positive thymocytes via TNF-alpha. *Eur. J. Immunol*, 30, 2586-2592.

[47] Bouman, A., Moes, H., Heineman, M.J., de Leij, L.F., Faas, M.M. (2001) The immune response during the luteal phase of the ovarian cycle: increasing sensitivity of human monocytes to endotoxin. *Fertil Steril*, 76, 555-559.

[48] Berg, G., Ekerfelt, C., Hammar, M., Lindgren, R., Matthiesen, L. Ernerudh, J. (2002) Cytokine changes in postmenopausal women treated with estrogens: a placebo-controlled study. *Am. J. Reprod. Immunol*, 48, 63-69.

[49] Brooks-Asplund, E.M., Tupper, C.E., Daun, J.M., Kenney, W.L. Cannon, J.G. (2002) Hormonal modulation of interleukin-6, tumor necrosis factor and associated receptor secretion in postmenopausal women. *Cytokine*, 19, 193-200.

[50] Ershler, W.B., Keller, E.T. (2000) Age-associated increased interleukin-6 gene expression, late-life diseases, and frailty. *Annu. Rev. Med*, 51, 245-270.

[51] Matalka, K.Z. (2003) The effect of estradiol, but not progesterone, on the production of cytokines in stimulated whole blood, is concentration-dependent. *Neuroendocrinol. Lett*, 24, 185-191.

[52] Majumder, B., Biswas, R., Chattopadhyay, U. (2002) Evaluation of an immunochemical fecal occult blood test with automated reading in screening for colorectal cancer in a general average-risk population. *Int. J. Cancer*, 97, 493-496.

[53] Kyurkchiev, D., Ivanova-Todorova, E., Hayrabedyan, S., Altankova, I., Kyurkchiev, S. (2007) Female sex steroid hormones modify some regulatory properties of monocyte-derived dendritic cells. *Am. J. Reprod. Immunol*, 58, 425-33.

[54] Paharkova-Vatchkova, V., Maldonado, R., Kovats, S. (2004) Estrogen preferentially promotes the differentiation of CD11c+ CD11b(intermediate) dendritic cells from bone marrow precursors. *J. Immunol*, 172, 1426.

[55] Jara, L.J., Benitez, G., Medina, G. (2008) Prolactin, dendritic cells, and systemic lupus erythematosus. *Autoimmun. Rev*, 7, 251-5.

[56] Matera, L., Mori, M., Galetto, A. (2001) Effect of prolactin on the antigen presenting function of monocyte-derived dendritic cells. *Lupus*, 10, 728-734.

[57] Molloy, E.J., O'Neill, A.J., Grantham, J.J., Sheridan-Pereira, M., Fitzpatrick, J.M., Webb, D.W., Watson, R.W. (2003) Sex-specific alterations in neutrophil apoptosis: the role of estradiol and progesterone. *Blood*, 102, 2653-2659.

[58] Bekesi, G., Kakucs, R., Varbiro, S., Racz, K., Sprintz, D., Feher, J., Szekacs, B. (2000) In vitro effects of different steroid hormones on superoxide anion production of human neutrophil granulocytes. *Steroids*, 65, 889-894.

[59] Cassidy, R.A. (2003) Influence of steroids on oxidant generation in activated human granulocytes and mononuclear leukocytes. *Shock*, 20, 85-90.

[60] Yovel, G., Shakhar, K., Ben Eliyahu, S. (2001) The effects of sex, menstrual cycle, and oral contraceptives on the number and activity of natural killer cells. *Gynecol. Oncol*, 81, 254-262.

[61] Grimaldi, C.M., Cleary, J., Dagtas, A.S., Moussai, D., Diamond, B. (2002) Estrogen alters thresholds for B cell apoptosis and activation. *J. Clin. Invest*, 109, 1625-1633.

[62] Medina, K.L., Strasser, A. Kincade, P.W. (2000) Estrogen influences the differentiation, proliferation, and survival of early B-lineage precursors. *Blood*, 95, 2059-2067.

[63] Kincade, P., Medina, K.L., Payne, K.J., Rossi, M.I., Tudor, K.S., Yamashita, Y. et al. (2000) Early B-lymphocyte precursors and their regulation by sex steroids. *Immunol. Rev*, 175, 128-137.

[64] Grimaldi, C., Michael, D., Diamond, B. (2001) Cutting edge: expansion and activation of a population of autoreactive marginal zone B cells in a model of estrogen-induced lupus. *J. Immunol*, 167, 1886-1890.

[65] Kamada, M., Irahara, M., Maegawa, M., Yasui, T., Yamano, S., Yamada, M., Tezuka, M., Kasai, Y., Deguchi, K., Ohmoto, Y. (2001) B cell subsets in postmenopausal women and the effect of hormone replacement therapy. *Maturitas*, 37, 173-179.

[66] Peeva, E., Michael, D., Cleary, J., Rice, J., Chen, X., Diamond, B. (2003) Prolactin modulates the naive B cell repertoire. *J. Clin. Invest*, 111, 275-283.

[67] Kochendoerfer, S., Krishnan, N., Buckley, D., Buckley, A. (2003) Prolactin regulation of Bcl-2 family members: increased expression of bcl-xL but not mcl-1 or bad in Nb2-T cells. *J. Endocrinol*, 178, 265-273.

[68] Thurmond, T.S., Murante, F.G., Staples, J.E., Silverstone, A.E., Korach, K.S., Gasiewicz, T.A. (2000) Role of estrogen receptor alpha in hematopoietic stem cell development and B lymphocyte maturation in the male mouse. *Endocrinology*, 141, 2309-2318.

[69] Medina, K.L., Garrett, K.P., Thompson, L.F., Rossi, M.I., Payne, K.J., Kincade, P.W. (2001) Identification of very early lymphoid precursors in bone marrow and their regulation by estrogen. *Nat. Immunol*, 2, 718-724.

[70] Grimaldi, C.M., Cleary, J., Dagtas, A.S., Moussai, D., Diamond, B. (2002) Estrogen alters thresholds for B cell apoptosis and activation. *J. Clin. Invest*, 109, 1625-1633.

[71] Kocar, I.H., Yesilova, Z., Ozata, M., Turan, M., Sengul, A., Ozdemir I. (2000) The effect of testosterone replacement treatment on immunological features of patients with Klinefelter's syndrome. *Clin. Exp. Immunol*, 121, 448-452.

[72] Yesilova, Z., Ozata, M., Kocar, I.H., Turan, M., Pekel, A., Sengul, A., Ozdemir, I.C. (2000) The effects of gonadotropin treatment on the immunological features of male patients with idiopathic hypogonadotropic hypogonadism. *J. Clin. Endocrinol. Metab*, 85, 66-70.

[73] Clowes, J.A., Riggs, B.L., Khosla, S. (2005) The role of the immune system in the pathophysiology of osteoporosis. *Immunol. Rev*, 208, 207-227.

[74] Weitzmann, M.N., Pacifici, R. (2005) The role of T lymphocytes in bone metabolism. *Immunol. Rev*, 208, 154-168.

[75] Teitelbaum, S.L. (2004) Postmenopausal osteoporosis, T cells, and immune dysfunction. *Proc. Natl. Acad. Sci. USA*, 101, 16711-2.

[76] Rifas, L., Arackal, S. (2003)T cells regulate the expression of matrix metalloproteinase in human osteoblasts via a dual mitogen-activated protein kinase mechanism. *Arthritis Rheum*, 48, 993-1001.

[77] Manolagas, S.C. (2000) Birth and death of bone cells: basic regulatory mechanisms and implications for the pathogenesis and treatment of osteoporosis. *Endocr. Rev*, 21, 115-137.

[78] Menaa, C., Kurihara, N., Roodman, G.D. (2000) CFU-GM-derived cells form osteoclasts at a very high efficiency. *Biochem. Biophys. Res. Commun*, 267, 943-946.

[79] Siggelkow, H., Eidner, T., Lehmann, G., Viereck, V., Raddarz, D., Munzel, U., et al. (2003) Cytokines, osteoprotegerin, and RANKL in vitro and histomorphometric indices of bone turnover in patients with different bone diseases. *J. Bone Miner. Res*, 18, 529-538.

[80] Teitelbaum, S.L. (2000) Bone resorption by osteoclasts. *Science*, 289, 1504-1508.

[81] Romas, E., Gillespie, M.T., Martin, T.J. (2002) Involvement of receptor activator of NFkappaB ligand and tumor necrosis factor-alpha in bone destruction in rheumatoid arthritis. *Bone*, 30, 340-346.

[82] Khosla, S. (2001) Minireview: the OPG/RANKL/RANK system. *Endocrinology*, 142, 5050-5055.

[83] Lam, J., Takeshita, S., Barker, J.E., Kanagawa, O. (2000) TNF-alpha induces osteoclastogenesis by direct stimulation of macrophages exposed to permissive levels of RANK ligand. *J. Clin. Invest*, 106, 1481-1488.

[84] Nanes, M.S. (2003) Tumor necrosis factor-alpha: molecular and cellular mechanisms in skeletal pathology. *Gene*, 321, 1-15.

[85] Wei, S., Kitaura, H., Zhou, P., Ross, F.P., Teitelbaum, S.L. (2005) IL-1 mediates TNF-induced osteoclastogenesis. *J. Clin. Invest*, 115, 282-290.

[86] Takayanagi, H., Ogasawara, K., Hida, S., Chiba, T., Murata, S., Sato, K., Takaoka, A., Yokochi, T., Oda, H., Tanaka, K., Nakamura, K., Taniguchi, T. (2000) T-cell-mediated

regulation of osteoclastogenesis by signalling cross-talk between RANKL and IFN-gamma. *Nature*, 408, 600-605.

[87] Arron, J.R., Choi, Y. (2000) Bone versus immune system. *Nature*, 408, 535-536.

[88] Wu, H., Arron, J.R. (2003) TRAF6, a molecular bridge spanning adaptive immunity, innate immunity and osteoimmunology. *BioEssays*, 25, 1096-1105.

[89] Scheidt-Nave, C., Bismar, H., Leidig-Bruckner, G., Woitge, H., Seibel, M.J., Ziegler, R., Pfeilschifter, J. (2001) Serum interleukin 6 is a major predictor of bone loss in women specific to the first decade past menopause. *J. Clin. Endocrinol. Metab*, 86, 2032-2042.

[90] Ferrari, S.L., Ahn-Luong, L., Garnero, P., Humphries, S.E., Greenspan, S.L. (2003) Two promoter polymorphisms regulating interleukin-6 gene expression are associated with circulating levels of C-reactive protein and markers of bone resorption in postmenopausal women. *J. Clin. Endocrinol. Metab*, 88, 255-259.

[91] Schett, G., Kiechl, S., Redlich, K., Oberhollenzer, F., Weger, S., Egger, G., Mayr, A., Jocher, J., Xu, Q., Pietschmann, P., Teitelbaum, S., Smolen J., Willeit, J. Soluble RANKL and risk of nontraumatic fracture. (2004) *JAMA*, 291, 1108-1113.

[92] Armour, K.J., Armour, K.E., van't Hof, R.J., Reid, D.M., Wei, X.Q., Liew, F.Y., et al. (2001) Activation of the inducible nitric oxide synthase pathway contributes to inflammation-induced osteoporosis by suppressing bone formation and causing osteoblast apoptosis. *Arthritis Rheum*, 44, 2790-2796.

[93] Abu-Amer Y. (2001) IL-4 abrogates osteoclastogenesis through STAT6-dependent inhibition of NF-kappaB. *J. Clin. Invest*, 107, 1375-1385.

[94] Ross, F.P. (2003) Interleukin 7 and estrogen-induced bone loss. *Trends Endocrinol. Metab*, 14, 147-149.

[95] Horwood, N.J., Elliott, J., Martin, T.J., Gillespie, M.T. (2001) IL-12 alone and in synergy with IL-18 inhibits osteoclast formation in vitro. *J Immunol*, 166, 4915-4921.

[96] Shi, Y., Massague, J. (2003) Mechanisms of TGF-beta signaling from cell membrane to the nucleus. *Cell*, 113, 685-700.

[97] Joseph, C., Kenny, A.M., Taxel, P., Lorenzo, J.A., Duque, G., Kuchel, G.A. (2005) Role of endocrine-immune dysregulation in osteoporosis, sarcopenia, frailty and fracture risk. *Mol. Aspects Med*, 26, 181-201.

[98] Marti, A., Marcos, A., Martinez, J.A. (2001) Obesity and immune function relationships. *Obes. Rev*, 2, 131-140.

[99] Coppack, S.W. (2001) Pro-inflammatory cytokines and adipose tissue. *Proc. Nutr. Soc.* 60, 349-356.

[100] Dixit, V.D., Taub, D.D. (2005) Ghrelin and immunity: a young player in an old field. *Exp. Gerontol*, 40, 900-910.

[101] Charriere, G., Cousin, B., Andre, M., Bacou, F., Pnecaud, L., Casteilla, L. (2003) Preadipocyte conversion to macrophage. Evidence of plasticity. *J. Biol. Chem*, 278, 9850-9855.

[102] Saillan-Barreau, C., Cousin, B., Andre, M., Villena, P., Casteilla, L., Penicaud, L. (2003) Human adipose cells as candidates in defense and tissue remodeling phenomena. *Biochem. Biophys. Res. Commun*, 309, 502-505.

[103] Yang, H., Youm, Y.H., Vandanmagsar, B., Rood, J., Kumar, K.G., Butler, A.A., Dixit, V.D. (2009) Obesity accelerates thymic aging. *Blood*, 114, 3803-3812.

[104] Kershaw, E.E., Flier, J.S. (2004) Adipose tissue as an endocrine organ. *J. Clin. Endocrinol. Metab*, 89, 2548-2556.

[105] Dixit, V.D., Mielenz, M., Taub, D.D., Parvizi, N. (2003) Leptin induces growth hormone secretion from peripheral blood mononuclear cells via a protein kinase C- and nitric oxide-dependent mechanism. *Endocrinology*, 144, 5595-5603.

[106] Otero, M., Lago, R., Gomez, R., Dieguez, C., Lago, F., Gomez-Reino, J., Gualillo, O. (2006) Towards a pro-inflammatory and immunomodulatory emerging role of leptin. *Rheumatology*, 45, 944-950.

[107] Tilg, H., Moschen, A.R. (2006) Adipocytokines: mediators linking adipose tissue, inflammation and immunity. *Nat. Rev. Immunol*, 6, 772-783.

[108] Farooqi, S., Matarese, G., Lord, G.M., Keogh, J.M., Lawrence, E., Agwu, C., Sanna, V., Jebb, S.A., Perna, F., Fontana, S., Lechler, R.I., DePaoli, A.M., O'Rahilly, S. (2002) Beneficial effects of leptin on obesity, T cell hyporesponsiveness, and neuroendocrine/metabolic dysfunction of human congenital leptin deficiency. *J. Clin. Invest*, 110, 1093-1103.

[109] Zarkesh-Esfahani, H., Pockley, G., Metcalfe, R.A., Bidlingmaier M, Wu Z, Ajami A, Weetman AP, Strasburger CJ, Ross RJ. (2001) High-dose leptin activates human leukocytes via receptor expression on monocytes. *J. Immunol*, 167, 4593-4599.

[110] Mancuso, P., Canetti, C., Gottschalk, A., Tithof, P.K., Peters-Golden, M. (2004) Leptin augments alveolar macrophage leukotriene synthesis by increasing phospholipase activity and enhancing group IVC iPLA2 (cPLA2gamma) protein expression. *Am. J. Physiol. Lung Cell Mol. Physiol*, 287, L497-502.

[111] Dixit, V.D., Schaffer, E.M., Pyle, R.S., Collins, G.D., Sakthivel, S.K., Palaniappan, R., Lillard Jr, J.W., Taub, D.D. (2004) Ghrelin inhibits leptin- and activation-induced proinflammatory cytokine expression by human monocytes and T cells. *J. Clin. Invest*, 114, 57-66.

[112] Raso, G.M., Pacilio, M., Esposito, E., Coppola, A., Di Carlo, R., Meli, R. (2002) Leptin potentiates IFN-gamma-induced expression of nitric oxide synthase and cyclo-oxygenase-2 in murine macrophage J774A.1. *Br. J. Pharmacol*, 137, 799-804.

[113] Fantuzzi, G., Faggioni, R. (2000) Leptin in the regulation of immunity, inflammation, and hematopoiesis. *J. Leukoc. Biol*, 68, 437-446.

[114] Hick, R.W., Gruver, A.L., Ventevogel, M.S., Haynes, B.F., Sempowski, G.D. (2006) Leptin selectively augments thymopoiesis in leptin deficiency and lipopolysaccharide-induced thymic atrophy. *J. Immunol*, 177, 169-176.

[115] Guzik, T.J., Mangalat, D., Korbut, R. (2006) Adipocytokines - novel link between inflammation and vascular function? *J. Physiol. Pharmacol*, 57, 505-528.

[116] Moore S.I., Huffnagle, G.B., Chen, G.H., White, E.S., Mancuso, P. (2003) Leptin modulates neutrophil phagocytosis of Klebsiella pneumoniae. *Infect Immun*, 71, 4182-4185.

[117] La Cava, A., Matarese, G. (2004) The weight of leptin in immunity. *Nat. Rev. Immunol*, 4, 371-379.

[118] Caldefie-Chezet, F., Poulin, A., Vasson, M.P. (2003) Leptin regulates functional capacities of polymorphonuclear neutrophils. *Free Radic. Res*, 37, 809-814.

[119] Park S, Rich J, Hanses F, Lee JC. (2009) Defects in innate immunity predispose C57BL/6J-Leprdb/Leprdb mice to infection by Staphylococcus aureus. *Infect Immun*, 77, 1008-1014.

[120] Tian, Z., Sun, R., Wei, H., Gao, B. (2002) Impaired natural killer (NK) cell activity in leptin receptor deficient mice: leptin as a critical regulator in NK cell development and activation. *Biochem. Biophys. Res. Commun*, 298, 297-302.

[121] Sanna, V., Di Giacomo, A, La Cava, A., Lechler, R.I., Fontana, S., Zappacosta, S., Matarese, G. (2003) Leptin surge precedes onset of autoimmune encephalomyelitis and correlates with development of pathogenic T cell responses. *J. Clin. Invest*, 111, 241-250.

[122] Matarese, G., Sanna, V., Lechler, R.I., Sarvetnick, N., Fontana, S., Zappacosta, S., La Cava, A. (2002) Leptin accelerates autoimmune diabetes in female NOD mice. *Diabetes*, 51, 1356-1361.

[123] Wolf, A.M., Wolf, D., Rumpold, H., Enrich, B., Tilg, H. (2004) Adiponectin induces the anti-inflammatory cytokines IL-10 and IL-1RA in human leukocytes. *Biochem. Biophys. Res. Commun*, 323, 630-635.

[124] Maeda, N., Shimomura, I., Kishida, K., Nishizawa, H., Matsuda, M., Nagaretani, H., Furuyama, N., Kondo, H., Takahashi, M., Arita, Y., Komuro, R., Ouchi, N., Kihara, S., Tochino, Y., Okutomi, K., Horie, M., Takeda, S., Aoyama, T., Funahashi, T., Matsuzawa, Y. (2002) Diet-induced insulin resistance in mice lacking adiponectin/ACRP30. *Nat. Med*, 8, 731-737.

[125] Yamaguchi, N., Argueta, J.G., Masuhiro, Y., Kagishita, M., Nonaka, K., Saito, T., Hanazawa, S., Yamashita, Y. (2005) Adiponectin inhibits Toll-like receptor family-induced signaling. *FEBS Lett*, 579, 6821-6826.

[126] Kim, K.Y., Kim, J.K., Han, S.H., Lim, J.S., Kim, K.I., Cho, D.H., Lee, M.S., Lee, J.H., Yoon, D.Y., Yoon, S.R., Chung, J.W., Choi, I., Kim, E., Yang, Y. (2006) Adiponectin is a negative regulator of NK cell cytotoxicity. *J. Immunol*, 176, 5958-5964.

[127] Yokota, T., Meka, C.S., Kouro, T., Medina, K.L., Igarashi, H., Takahashi, M., Oritani, K., Funahashi, T., Tomiyama, Y., Matsuzawa, Y., Kincade, P.W. (2003) Adiponectin, a fat cell product, influences the earliest lymphocyte precursors in bone marrow cultures by activation of the cyclooxygenase-prostaglandin pathway in stromal cells. *J. Immunol*, 171, 5091-5099.

[128] Kaser, S., Kaser, A., Sandhofer, A., Ebenbichler, C.F., Tilg, H., Patsch, J.R. (2003) Resistin messenger-RNA expression is increased by proinflammatory cytokines in vitro. *Biochem. Biophys. Res. Commun*, 309, 286-290.

[129] Silswal, N., Singh, A.K., Aruna, B., Mukhopadhyay, S., Ghosh, S., Ehtesham, N.Z. (2005) Human resistin stimulates the pro-inflammatory cytokines TNF-alpha and IL-12 in macrophages by NF-kappaB-dependent pathway. *Biochem. Biophys. Res. Commun*, 334, 1092-1101.

[130] Tilg, H., Moschen, A.R. (2006) Adipocytokines: mediators linking adipose tissue, inflammation and immunity. *Nat. Rev. Immunol*, 6, 772-83.

[131] Matarese, G., Mantzoros, C., La Cava, A. (2007) Leptin and adipocytokines: bridging the gap between immunity and atherosclerosis. *Curr. Pharma Design*, 13, 3676-3680.

[132] Moschen, A.R., Kaser, A., Enrich, B., Mosheimer, B., Theurl, M., Niederegger, H., Tilg, H. (2007) Visfatin, an adipocytokine with proinflammatory and immunomodulating properties. *J. Immunol*, 178, 1748-58.

[133] Cianflone, K., Xia, Z., Chen, L.Y. (2003) Critical review of acylation-stimulating protein physiology in humans and rodents. *Biochim. Biophys. Acta*, 1609, 127-143.

[134] Gnanapavan, S., Kola, B., Bustin, S.A., Morris, D.G., McGee, P., Fairclough, P., Bhattacharya, S., Carpenter R., Grossman, A.B., Korbonits, M. (2002) The tissue distribution of the mRNA of ghrelin and subtypes of its receptor, GHS-R, in humans. *J. Clin. Endocrinol. Metab*, 87, 2988.

[135] Xia, Q., Pang, W., Pan, H., Zheng, Y., Kang, J.S., Zhu, S.G. (2004) Effects of ghrelin on the proliferation and secretion of splenic T lymphocytes in mice. *Regul. Pept*, 122, 173-178.

[136] Matsuki, T., Horai, R., Sudo, K., Iwakura, Y. (2003) IL-1 plays an important role in lipid metabolism by regulating insulin levels under physiological conditions. *J. Exp. Med*, 198, 877-888.

[137] Juge-Aubry, C.E., Somm, E., Giusti, V., Pernin, A., Chicheportiche, R., Verdumo, C., Rohner-Jeanrenaud, F., Burger, D., Dayer, J.M., Meier, C.A. (2003) Adipose tissue is a major source of interleukin-1 receptor antagonist: upregulation in obesity and inflammation. *Diabetes*, 52, 1104-1110.

[138] Fernandez-Real, J.M., Ricart, W. (2003) Insulin resistance and chronic cardiovascular inflammatory syndrome. *Endocr. Rev*, 24, 278-301.

[139] Fain, J.N., Madan, A.K., Hiler, M.L., Cheema, P., Bahouth, S.W. (2004) Comparison of the release of adipokines by adipose tissue, adipose tissue matrix, and adipocytes from visceral and subcutaneous abdominal adipose tissues of obese humans. *Endocrinology*, 145, 2273-2282.

[140] Wajchenberg, B.L. (2000) Subcutaneous and visceral adipose tissue: their relation to the metabolic syndrome. *Endocr. Rev*, 21, 697-738.

[141] Wallenius, V., Wallenius, K., Ahren, B., Rudling, M., Carlsten, H., Dickson, S.L., Ohlsson, C., Jansson, J.O. (2002) Interleukin-6-deficient mice develop mature-onset obesity. *Nat. Med*, 8, 75-79.

[142] Hotamisligil, G.S. (2003) Inflammatory pathways and insulin action. *Int. J. Obes. Relat. Metab. Disord*, 27, S53-55.

[143] Ruan, H., Lodish, H.F. (2003) Insulin resistance in adipose tissue: direct and indirect effects of tumor necrosis factor-alpha. *Cytokine Growth Factor Rev*, 14, 447-455.

[144] Warne, J.P., (2003), Tumour necrosis factor alpha: a key regulator of adipose tissue mass. *J. Endocrinol*, 177, 351-355.

[145] Fruhbeck, G., Gómez-Ambrosi, J., Muruzábal, F.J., Burrell, M.A. (2001) The adipocyte: a model for integration of endocrine and metabolic signaling in energy metabolism regulation. *Am. J. Physiol. Endocrinol. Metab*, 280, E827-847.

[146] Ruan, H., Miles, P.D., Ladd, C.M., Ross, K., Golub, T.R., Olefsky, J.M., Lodish, H.F. (2002) Profiling gene transcription in vivo reveals adipose tissue as an immediate target of tumor necrosis factor-alpha: implications for insulin resistance. *Diabetes*, 51, 3176-3188.

[147] Arsenijevic, D., Garcia, I., Vesin, C., Vesin, D., Arsenijevic, Y., Seydoux, J., Girardier, L., Ryffel, B., Dulloo, A., Richard, D. (2000) Differential roles of tumor necrosis factor-alpha and interferon-gamma in mouse hypermetabolic and anorectic responses induced by LPS. *Eur. Cytokine Netw*, 11, 662-668.

[148] Wellen, K.E., Hotamisligil, G.S. (2003) Obesity-induced inflammatory changes in adipose tissue. *J Clin Invest*, 112, 1785-1788.

[149] Takahashi, K., Mizuarai, S., Araki, H., Mashiko, S., Ishihara, A., Kanatani, A., Itadani, H., Kotani, H. (2003) Adiposity elevates plasma MCP-1 levels leading to the increased CD11b-positive monocytes in mice. *J. Biol. Chem*, 278, 46654-46660.

[150] Sartipy, P., Loskutoff, D.J. (2003) Monocyte chemoattractant protein 1 in obesity and insulin resistance. *Proc. Natl. Acad. Sci. USA*, 100, 7265-7270.

[151] Gerhardt, C.C., Romero, I.A., Cancello, R., Camoin, L., Strosberg, A.D. (2001) Chemokines control fat accumulation and leptin secretion by cultured human adipocytes. *Mol. Cell Endocrinol*, 175, 81-92.

[152] Klein, J.R. (2006) The immune system as a regulator of thyroid hormone activity. *Exp. Biol. Med*, 231, 229-236.

[153] Bagriacik, E.U., Zhou, Q., Wang, H.C., Klein, J. (2001) Rapid and transient reduction in circulating thyroid hormones following systemic antigen priming: implications for functional collaboration between dendritic cells and thyroid. *Cell Immunol*, 212, 92-100.

[154] Klein, J.R., Wang, H.C. (2004) Characterization of a novel set of resident intrathyroidal bone marrow-derived hematopoietic cells: potential for immune-endocrine interactions in thyroid homeostasis. *J. Exp. Biol*, 207, 55–65.

[155] Wang, H.C., Dragoo, J., Zhou, Q., Klein, J.R. (2003) An intrinsic thyrotropin-mediated pathway of TNF-alpha production by bone marrow cells. *Blood*, 101, 119–123.

[156] Bagriacik, E.U., Klein, J.R. (2000) The thyrotropin (thyroid-stimulating hormone) receptor is expressed on murine dendritic cells and on a subset of CD45RBhigh lymph node T cells: functional role for thyroid-stimulating hormone during immune activation. *J. Immunol*, 164, 6158–6165.

[157] Beigneux, A.P., Moser, A.H., Shigenaga, J.K., Grunfeld, C., Feingold, K.R. (2003) Sick euthyroid syndrome is associated with decreased TR expression and DNA binding in mouse liver. *Am. J. Physiol. Endocrinol. Metab*, 284, E228–236.

[158] Fakete, C., Singru, P.S., Sarkar, S., Rand, W.M., Lechan, R.M. (2005) Ascending brainstem pathways are not involved in lipopolysaccharide-induced suppression of thyrotropin-releasing hormone gene expression in the hypothalamic paraventricular nucleus. *Endocrinology*, 146, 1357–1363.

[159] Weetman, A.P. (2004) Cellular immune responses in autoimmune thyroid disease. *Clin. Endocrinol*, 61, 405–413.

[160] Collins, J., Gough, S. (2002) Autoimmunity in thyroid disease. *Eur. J. Nucl. Med. Mol. Imaging*, 29, S417–424.

[161] Weetman, A.P. (2001) Determinants of autoimmune thyroid disease. *Nat. Immunol*, 2, 769–770.

[162] Sakaguchi, S., Sakaguchi, N., Shimizu, J., Yamazaki, S., Sakihama, T., Itoh, et al. (2001) Immunologic tolerance maintained by CD25+ CD4+ regulatory T cells: their common role in controlling autoimmunity, tumor immunity, and transplantation tolerance. *Immunol. Rev*, 182, 18–32.

[163] Watanabe, M., Yamamoto, N., Maruoka, H., Matsuzuka, F., Miyauchi, A., Iwatani, Y. (2003) Relation of CD30 molecules on T-cell subsets to the severity of autoimmune thyroid disease. *Thyroid*, 13, 259–263.

[164] Nagayama, Y., Mizuguchi, H., Hayakawa, T., Niwa, M., McLachlan, S.M., Rapoport, B. (2003) Prevention of autoantibody-mediated Graves'-like hyperthyroidism in mice with IL-4, a Th2 cytokine. *J. Immunol*, 170, 3522–3527.

[165] Dogan, R.-N.E., Vasu, C., Holterman, M.J., Prabhakar, B.S. (2003) Absence of IL-4, and not suppression of the Th2 response, prevents development of experimental autoimmune Graves' disease. *J. Immunol*, 170, 2195–2204.

[166] De Metz, J., Romijn, J.I., Endert, E., Crossmit, E.P., Sauerwein, H.P. (2000) Administration of interferon-gamma in healthy subjects does not modulate thyroid hormone metabolism. *Thyroid*, 10, 87–91.

[167] Armengol, M.-P., Cardoso-Schmidt, C.B., Fernández, M., Ferrer, X., Pujol-Borrell, R., Juan, M. (2003) Chemokines determine local lymphoneogenesis and a reduction of circulating CXCR4+ T and CCR7 B and T lymphocytes in thyroid autoimmune diseases. *J. Immunol*, 170, 6320–6328.

[168] Takiyama, Y., Miyokawa, N., Tokusashi, Y., Ito, K., Kato, S., Kimura, S., et al. (2002) Thyroid-stimulating hormone induces interleukin-18 gene expression in FRTL-5 cells: immunohistochemical detection of interleukin-18 in autoimmune thyroid disease. *Thyroid*, 12, 935–943.

[169] Klecha, A.J., Arcos, M.L.B., Frick, L., Genaro, A.M., Cremaschi, G. (2008) Immune-endocrine interactions in autoimmune thyroid diseases. *Neuroimmunomodulation*, 15, 68–75.

[170] Allahabadia, A., Heward, J.M., Nithiyananthan, R., Gibson, S.M., Reuser, T.T., Dodson, P.M., et al. (2001) MHC class II region, CTLA4 gene, and ophthalmopathy in patients with Graves' disease. *Lancet*, 358, 984–985.

[171] Simmonds, M.J., Howson, J.M., Heward, J.M., Carr-Smith, J., Franklyn, J.A., Todd, J.A., et al. (2007) A novel and major association of HLA-C in Graves' disease that eclipses the classical HLA-DRB1 effect. *Hum. Mol. Genet*, 16, 2149–2153.

[172] Takara, M., Komiya, I., Kinjo, Y., Tomoyose, T., Yamashiro, S., Akamine, H. (2000) Association of CTLA-4 gene A/G polymorphism in Japanese type 1 diabetic patients with younger age of onset and autoimmune thyroid disease. *Diabetes Care*, 23, 975–978.

[173] Tomer, Y., Greenberg, D.A., Barbesino, G., Concepcion, E., Davies, T.F. (2001) CTLA-4 and not CD28 is a susceptibility gene for thyroid autoantibody production. *J. Clin. Endocrinol. Metab*, 86, 1687–1693.

[174] Hunt, P.J., Marshall, S.E., Weetman, A.P., Bell, J.I., Wass, J.A., Welsh, K.I. (2000) Cytokine gene polymorphisms in autoimmune thyroid disease. *J. Clin. Endocrinol. Metab*, 85, 1984–1988.

[175] Heward, J.M., Nithiyananthan, R., Allahabadia, A., Gibson, S., Franklyn, J.A., Gough, S.C., (2001) No association of an interleukin 4 gene promoter polymorphism with Graves' disease in the United Kingdom. *J. Clin. Endocrinol. Metab*, 86, 3861–3863.

[176] Jacobson, E.M., Tomer, Y. (2007) The CD40, CTLA-4, thyroglobulin, TSH receptor, and PTPN22 gene quintet and its contribution to thyroid autoimmunity: back to the future. *J. Autoimmun*, 28, 85–98.

[177] Ciampolillo, A., Guastamacchia, E., Amati, L., Magrone, T., Munno, I., Jirillo, et al. (2003) Modifications of the immune responsiveness in patients with autoimmune thyroiditis: evidence for a systemic immune alteration. *Curr. Pharm. Des*, 9, 1946–19450.

[178] Klecha, A.J., Genaro, A.M., Lysionek, A.E., Caro, R.A., Coluccia, G.A., Cremaschi, G.A. (2000) Experimental evidence pointing to the bidirectional interaction between the immune system and the thyroid axis. *Int. J. Immunopharmacol*, 22, 491–500.

[179] Klecha, A.J., Genaro, A.M., Gorelik, G., Barreiro, Arcos, M.L., Silberman, D.M., et al. (2006) Integrative study of hypothalamus-pituitary-thyroid-immune system interaction: thyroid hormone-mediated modulation of lymphocyte activity through the protein kinase C signaling pathway. *J. Endocrinol*, 189, 45–55.

In: Immunology in Clinic Practice
Editor: Cagatay Oktenli, pp. 137-155
ISBN 978-1-60876-644-4


*Chapter 8*

# IMMUNOLOGY IN HEMATOLOGY: RECENT ADVANCES

***Özkan Sayan*[1] *and M. Hakan Terekeci*[2]**
1. Division of Hematology,
GATA Haydarpasa Training Hospital, Istanbul, Turkey
2. Division of Internal Medicine,
GATA Haydarpasa Training Hospital, Istanbul, Turkey

## ABSTRACT

Immunohematology is a scientific scope that deals with and reveals particularly erythrocytes, immunological incidents regarding blood cells and blood groups, with special emphasis on antigen-antibody reactions, connection and interaction thereof with diseases. The specialist working in this scope is named immunohematologist. The term 'blood cell' refers to antigens made up of various gene alleles which are controlled by a locus found on the erythrocytes. Many blood groups, such as ABO, have been revealed so far and they have also been genetically defined.

**Keywords:** Immunohematology; blood cells; blood group antigents; Rh antibodies; acute hemolytic transfusion reactions

## INTRODUCTION

ABO blood types compromise the fundamental system in the typing of the blood types [1]. All donor blood for transfusion is tested and labeled with the ABO group. The four main phenotypes are A, B, AB, and O, the latter indicating a lack of both A and B antigens. The sugars defining A and B antigens are added to carbohydrate chains carrying the H antigen, which is "invisible" by the A or B sugar. Thus group A or B erythrocytes appear to have less

H antigen than group O cells. However, H is found on all human erythrocytes except those in rare individuals of the $O_h$ (Bombay) phenotype.

## Blood Group Antigens

The identification of ABO blood group antigens has been one of the most significant steps in safe transfusion [2,3]. The studies conducted so far have revealed that various structures related to membrane in blood cells display antigenic characteristics that could form antibody response [4]. The number of blood group antigens identified serologically exceeds 600 [5].

The majority of such antigens are interrelated and they compose the blood group systems. 29 blood group systems among blood group antigens were described, and out of these 9 blood groups were approved the major group system by the International Society of Blood Transfusion (ISBT) in 2004 [6].

The biochemical structure of many blood group systems has been identified up until now. ABH, Lewis, P and I blood group antigens are in the carbonhydrate structure [7]. The ABO blood group system consists of four antigens (A, B, O and AB). These antigens are known as oligosaccharide antigens. The A and B antigens are mainly expressed on erythrocytes, but are also weakly expressed on platelets and endothelial cells. The genes of ABO blood group have been determined at chromosome locus 9 [8]. The AB and O genes are inherited according to Mendel's principles [9]. The antigens in multivalent carbonhydrate can directly synthesize antibody from B lymphocytes. This immune response leads to the formation of immunoglobulin M type (IgM) antibody [10]. The antibodies formed in this way are called isohemagglutinin. Sometimes IgG type antibodies may form with a high titer against carbonhydrate blood group antigens.

The bulk of knowledge regarding the chemical structures of blood group antigens like Rh, MNS, Kell, Lutheran, Kidd, Duffy and XG in the protein structure is relatively far less compared to that with carbonhydrate [11]. The most typical characteristic is that they form an immune response dependent on thymus [12]. Antigen specific helper leads to the formation of antibodies in the IgG structure from B lymphocytes through T lymphocytes. The IgG type antibodies generally cause extravascular hemolysis [13].

### ABO Blood Group System

There are three antigens in the ABO system [14-17]. These are A, B and H. The H antigen is found in all the blood groups of A, B and O [18]. It is defined as a carrying molecule for A and B antigens. The "O" letter in the O group is the first letter of the German word "ohne" which means "without" in English. It means without antigen, referring to the absence of the A and B antigens. The existence of strong reactive antibodies in serum against antigens not found on the erythrocyte surface is another characteristic of this group [19]. These two characteristics render the ABO system the most significant antigens in transfusion and tissue transplantation.

The antigens belonging to the ABO system are found as the membrane antigens in the following locations: on the surface of erythrocyte and platelets, vascular epithelium cells, epithelium cells like intestinal, cervical and glandula mammaria; in the dissolved form they are found in plasma, saliva, milk and feces [20].

These antigens belonging to ABO system are controlled at least by three gene locations as: a) H ve h; b) A1, A2, B ve O; c) Se and se. Each gene location is dependent from the others.

The most striking variant of ABH system is the Bombay phenotype [21]. They have no H antigens on the erythrocyte surface and high titer anti-H antibodies in their serum. Although some individuals have active A and B gene, the carrying H antigen molecule is not completed. For this reason, the enzyme cannot be synthesized yet the A or B genes in such individuals can be transferred to the next generation. In this way, A or B group children are bred by O group- Bombay phenotype parents. Some individuals do not have ABH antigens on the erythrocyte surface yet it is possible to detect ABH antigens in their secretions. These individuals can synthesize H type 1 glycoside transferase but cannot synthesize type 2 transferase. This phenotype is named “Para-Bombay”.

## Antibodies Belonging to ABO System

The developed antibodies belonging to ABO system are examined in two groups, which are natural and immune [22]. Both types occur as a result of immunization. Natural anti-A and anti-B antibodies are generally in the structure of IgM, on the other hand, immune anti-A and anti-B antibodies are in the structure of IgG, developing most frequently as a result of fetal-maternal hemorrhage. The immunogen in the naturally developing antibodies has bacterial source. Bacteria found in flora and blood group antigens have similarities. It is considered that the antigens in IgM structure developed against these bacteria form the natural antibodies identified as isohemagglutinin.

Anti-A, B antibodies found in the serums of the O group individuals yield agglutination both in A and B type erythrocytes, yet they cannot be differentiated as A and B through absorption techniques [23]. When retests are conducted with the “eluates” derived from the serums reacted with A cells, it is expected that they display reaction only with cells having A antigen. However, it is seen that they display reaction both with A cells and B cells once again. In addition, the saliva of A or B group secretors can inhibit both the A and B activity of this antibody.

Anti-Al antibodies display reaction with Al cells. B, O, A2 and A2B can be found in the serums of the individuals with Ax blood groups in varying amounts. Anti-H antibodies form a very strong agglutination with O cells but form a weaker one with A2 and A3 cells. The weakest agglutination is seen with Al and AIB cells. Anti-H is found in the serums of the individuals with Bombay type (Oh) blood group [24].

# Rh System

The antiserum, derived via the process of giving rabbits the erythrocytes taken from Macacus Rhesus monkeys, agglutinate 85% of the human erythrocytes [25]. This fact was first introduced by Landsteiner and Wiener, and the antigen was named Rh antigen. It was later understood that this D antigen with the highest antigenity, following A and B antigens.

## Rh Antigens

Rh system is one of the most complicated erythrocyte antigen systems, with more than 40 allele and variants defined [26-28]. The most important ones are the antigens controlled by three allele gen couples. Three different systems such as Fisher-Race, Wiener ve Rosenfield (digital) are used to name the antigens [26].

Fisher-Race name system is commonly used as it is easier and comprehensible. These three allele genes or isoantigens have been named as Cc, Dd and Ee. It is possible to form eight different haplotypes (gene complex) through the eight different combinations of these genes. Antibody developed against C, c, E, e ve D antigens can be shown in serum, and however, no antibody could be shown against the “d antigen”. Nevertheless, the existence of “d antigen” is accepted in cases where “D antigen” cannot be shown [27].

Since the strongest antigen in Rh system is D, erythrocytes agglutinated with anti-D are called “Rh positive”, those which are not agglutinated are called “Rh negative”. When one unit of Rh positive blood is delivered to Rh negative individuals, anti-D antibodies form in 70 % of these individuals. Yet, D antigen doesn’t always display a strong reaction. Stratton, in 1946, revealed the erythrocytes carrying weak D antigen. He defined this structure as “Du”. Argall'm, in 1953, named Anti-D antibody as "D-variant antigen" in an individual with Rh positive. Through Moore’s suggestion in 1953 the “weak-D antigen” definition was approved instead of Du antigen.

As for Weak-D and Variant-D, the replies of the following questions and clinical preventions are still controversial: 1- Whether the weak or variant D antige can form antibody response in a Rh negative individual, 2- Whether a fetus with weak or variant D can immunize a Rh negative mother, 3- Whether antibody response occurs if Rh positive blood is delivered to the recipient carrying weak or variant D antigen, and 4-Whether a mother with weak or variant D antigen can be immunized with Rh positive fetus. The existence of lacking / deficient antigenic epitopes in the variant D antigen forms the adequate requirements for the antibody response even if the possibility is low. For this reason, approaching such individual through blood banks is quite significant. That is why, polyclonal IgG type antiserum usage is recommended to avoid negative record and have DVI variant display in the donors. It is also suggested that two high avidity monoclonal anti-D grouping both for the donors and recipients should be administered [25].

## Rh Antibodies

Rh antibodies, except some exceptions like anti-Cw and anti-E, are antibodies in the structure of immune originated IgG; they do not form intravascular hemolysis. IgM or IgA type Rh antibodies are rare. Their existence can be best proven by albumin, enzim and Coombs tests. It is accepted that they occur mostly following fetal-maternal hemorrhage as they are scanned routinely before the transfusion. D antigen does not display dosage (reaction discrepancy due to level) but anti-C, anti-c, anti-E and anti-e antibodies often display dosage and form stronger aggluniation with homozygote cells compared to heterozygote cells.

## Other Red Cell Antigens

### *Lewis System*

Lewis antigens are synthesized in other tissues, most probably in the intestinal epithelium [29]. They are later absorbed in the erythrocyte surface. Lewis and ABH antigens are closely linked, coding Le gene (1-4) fucosiletransferase. The antibodies of Lewis system are anti-Le (a) and anti-Le (b) natural antibodies in the structure of IgM. Hemolytic transfusion reaction due to Anti-Le (a) has been reported but neonatal hemolytic disease does not occur as they cannot go beyond placenta because of their IgM structure. The Lewis substances in the serum are typed invitro. They can neutralize the antibodies invivo during the transfusion process.

### *Kell Blood Group System*

Kell Blood Groups System is a complicated blood group system [30]. The biochemistry of the antigens belonging to this system has not been clearly understood yet.

Kell antibodies can be shown invitro by Coombs, the existence of enzymes in the setting test does not exacerbate the reaction [31]. They can cause hemolytic transfusion reactions and neonatal hemolytic disease. The antigens belonging to Kell system have the second strongest structure, after D antigen in terms of antigenity other than A and B antigen.

### *Duffy System*

The frequency of antigens in Duffy system display distinctive differences in Caucasians and black race. In Caucasians two allele genes as Fya and Fyb are found.

The most frequently stored antibodies of Duffy system in the blood banks are Anti-Fya and Anti-Fyb. These antibodies with immune origin are in the IgG class and they can be found both in hemolytic transfusion reactions and neonatal hemolytic disease.

### *Kidd System*

As it is the case with other blood groups it is a system that does not have numerous antigens. It has tow allele genes: Jka and Jkb. The third gene is $Jk^3$ gene. Jka, Jkb and Jkajkb form the antigens of the Kidd system. They are not found in the leukocyte or platelets. The Jk (a-b-) phenotype is rarely seen and it is described by "silent allele" Jk gene derived from both parents.

Anti-Jka and anti-Jkb antibodies are in IgG structure and these antibodies are shown via Coombs test. They frequently display dosage. They should be treated with enzyme in order to detect them. Transfusion reactions and neonatal hemolytic disease due to Kidd antibodies are not encountered frequently.

***Lutheran System***

The exact structure of Lutheran antigens is not entirely or adequately known. There are at least 19 Lutheran antigens [32]. Lutheran antibodies cause transfusion reaction and neonatal hemolytic disease in rare cases.

***MNSs System***

MN antigens have been found on glycophorin A made up of 131 aminoacids and 16 oligosaccharides in the erythrocyte membrane [33].

Anti-M and anti-N antibodies are those found naturally in the serum with IgM strcuture [34]. Anti-S and anti-s are frequently in IgG structure; anti-U is always in IgG structure. Anti-M and anti-N react better in acid pH. The agglutination strength of Anti-M, anti-N and anti-S decrease with erythrocytes treated with enzyme. As Anti-s and anti-U are in IgG structure, their optimal reaction temperature is 37°C, for Anti-M and anti-N antibodies form reaction below 37°C. They can rarely have IgG structure and cause neonatal hemolytic disease in rare cases. However, when there is a hemolytic disease in such a case, this could have a severe course. Transfusion reactions and neonatal hemolytic disease related to anti-S, anti-s and anti-U have also been reported.

## Erythrocytes Antibodies

Antigen-oriented antibodies located on the surface of erythrocytes can be natural or immune, complete or incomplete, hot or cold. Besides, erythrocyte antibodies are divided into two groups: alloantibodies (isoantibodies) and autoantibodies.

### Natural and Immune Antibodies

Antibodies which are not formed as a result of a visible immunization oriented towards blood type antigens which are not found in one's own erythrocytes are called "natural" or "naturally-formed antibodies." Isohemaglutinins such as anti-A and anti-B in ABO system are some examples to this kind of antibodies. It is definitely impossible to know how natural antibodies are formed. These antibodies are not found in human body during birth. Cross reaction is supposed to be found between polysaccharid antigens of erythrocytes and certain bacteria in nature and virus antigens. Once a body encounters such antigens, it produces antibodies against what is not available in its own erythrocytes.

Natural antibodies are almost always oriented towards antigens in the carbohydrate structure of erythrocytes (e.g. ABH, MN, P, Lewis, I and i). They usually belong to IgM class. Therefore, they cannot pass through plasenta. Besides, they are usually complete antibodies and they enter into reaction with antigen at temperatures below ***37°C*** (optimum 4° ***C***) (cold antibodies).

Immune antibodies develop as a result of the sensitivity of a body by means of erythrocyte antigens which are not found in one's own erythrocytes. This immunization is under the responsibility of blood incompatibility between the mother and fetus (e.g. Rh incompatibility) or blood transfusion from wrong blood type (e.g. transfusion of blood from a person with Rh positive to the one with Rh negative).

Immune antibodies are oriented towards antigens found in the protein structure of erythrocytes (e.g. Rh, Kell, Kidd, Duffy). These antigens are also called "immunogenic antigens". In some cases it is possible that immune (unnatural) anti-A and anti-B antibodies related to ABO system develop (e.g. ABO incompatibility between the mother and fetus).

Immune antibodies are usually incomplete IgG class antibodies which enter into reaction best at ***37°C*** ("hot") and they can go through plasenta.

## Complete and Incomplete Antibodies

Erythrocyte antibodies are formed in vitro by means of agglutination. Antibodies which can aggregate erythrocytes in isotonic salty water environment are called "complete", and those which cannot aggregate are called "incomplete."

Ig molecules have at least two (as IgG in monomer structure has) or more connecting points (as IgM in pentamer form has) with antigen. Normally suspending erythrocytes have a negative electrostatic charge-cloud on their surface. This negative charge that moves two erythrocytes in opposite directions is called "zeta potential." Main factors which affect zeta potential are the features of erythrocyte membrane surface and the environment in which erythrocytes are found. An Ig molecule has to defeat repelling electrostatic power in order to lay a bridge between two erythrocytes. In the environment of isotonic water IgM, which is a large pentamer-shaped molecule, agglutinates erythrocytes easily defeating zeta potential. However, IgG cannot agglutinate erythrocytes in the same environment.

Natural antibodies and cold aglutinins are complete antibodies that belong to IgM class. Most immune antibodies and "hot" autoantibodies observed in autoimmune hemolytic anemia are "incomplete" antibodies that belong to IgG class.

It is necessary to refer to methods which will change zeta potential in order to maintain agglutination with incomplete antibodies as is the case in the process of erythrocytes with proteolytic enzymes that destroy membrane surface or the suspension of erythrocytes in the colloidal environment. Another method used in the fixatition of incomplete antibodies that cover the surface of erythrocytes is called Coombs (antiglobulin) test.

## Direct Coombs Test

Let us think of erythrocytes covered with IgG type incomplete antibodies. Erythrocytes cannot aggregate as these antibodies are not able to defeat zeta potential. If immune serum which contains antibodies against human IgG prepared from animals like rabbits is added to the environment, these anti-IgGs can help agglutination with IgGs on the surface of the erythrocytes building bridges. And such immune serum is called "Coombs (antiglobulin) serum."

Coombs serum is prepared by injecting human Igs to animals (rabbits) [35]. As it is possible to inject the entire globulin fraction of human serum- in this case what is obtained is polyvalent Coombs serum-, it is also possible to inject certain Ig fraction (IgG) or complement component (C3). Coombs serum which is obtained under this final environment are monospecific. For example, direct Coombs test in cold agglutinin disease gives positive results with anti-C3 serums.

Direct Coombs test is used in fixation of IgG class allo and autoantibodies which are adherent in vivo to erythrocytes. Direct Coombs is found to be positive in autoimmune hemolytic anemia with "hot" antibodies. The test which is made with cord blood erythrocytes is positive in the hemolytic disease of a new born resulting from Rh incompatibility.

Erythrocytes to be examined are washed away from their plasmas. Then they are incubated with Commbs serum. If aglutination occurs, the result is positive. This used to be done in tubes. Nowadays gel technology is used.

## Indirect Coombs Test

With this test incomplete antibodies which are not adherent to erythrocytes in patient serum are searched for. Indirect test is used in the prenatal track of pregnant women in Rh incompatibility, in the search for atypic antibodies in receiver serum before erythrocyte transfusions [36]. In some cases of autoimmune hemolytic anemia with "hot" antibodies, both direct Coombs and indirect test can be found to be positive. This symptom indicates the gravity of prognosis.

The patient serum to be examined is first incubated with O Rh (+) erythrocytes or erythrocytes whose antigens are known in the search for "atypic" antibodies. Incubation helps incomplete antibodies adhere to erythrocyctes. Later, erythrocytes are washed and compared with Coombs serum as it is the case in direct test.

Eryhtrocyte antibodies are divided into two as "hot" or "those which react at high temperatures" or "cold" or " those which react at low temperatures" according to the temperature of the environment where eryhtrocyte-antibody interaction develops. Hot antibodies show maximum reaction at normal body temperature (aroud 37° C). On the other hand, cold antibodies usually unite with erythrocytes at temperatures below 30°C and maximum 4° C When temperature increases, cold antibodies detach from erythrocytes again.

When thermal amplitude of a cold antibody matters, it means the utmost temperature (e.g. 30-31°C) at which that antibody can react with erythrocytes. The thermal amplitude of antibodies is especially important in terms of the weight and variety of clinical symptoms in cold agglutinin disease.

## Alloantibodies and Autoantibodies

Immune antibodies which develop as a result of sensitivity against erythrocyte antigens are divided into two: "alloantibodies" and "autoantibodies."

Different (allelic) antigens which are controlled by the same genetic locus in species (e.g human) are called "alloantigen". Antibodies which develop against these antigens are called alloantibodies. Alloantibody is the synonym of "isoantibody". Alloimmunization is at issue after incompatible blood transfusion and in feto-maternal blood incompatibility.

Autoantibodies are antibodies which develop against one's own antigens. They react together with erythrocyte antigens of almost all individuals of the same kind. Erythrocyte autoantibodies which can be "hot" and "cold" lead to hemolytic anemia. Erythrocyte autoantibodies rarely develop as a result of medicine allergies.

Erythrocyte autoantibodies have an antigenic specificity. Hot autoantibodies (IgG) are usually oriented towards antigens of Rh system. Cold aglutinins (IgM) in autoimmune hemolytic anemia with cold antibodies usually bear a specificity of anti-I or anti-i. Donath-Landsteiner antibody (IgG) in proxysmal cold hemoglobinuris has a specificity of anti-P.

## The results of Erythrosite-Antibody Interaction

Erythrocyte-oriented antibodies lead to the demolishment of eryhtrocytes (immune hemolisis) using the following mechanisms [37].

### *1. Opsonic Adherence and Phagocytosis*

Monocytes and macrophages which are located in spleen and liver can catch and phagositize (opsonic adherence) Fc receptors and erythrocytes covered with IgG class antibodies. Hemolysis is then extravascular. As complement has C3b receptors against C3b component, erythrocytes covered with C3b can adhere in this way (immuno-adherence) and undergo phagocytosis.

Adherence may not always result in phagocytosis. Sometimes adherence is temporary. Meanwhile, macrophage tears off a bit of erythrocyte membrane and then the floating cell takes the form of spherocyte and keeps its integrity. Spherocytosis is a common symptom in autoimmune hemolytic anemia with hot antibodies. Antibodies leading to spherocytosis belong to IgG class (especially IgG1 and IgG3). As osmotic and mechanic fragility of spherocytes increases, the life span of spherocytes declines while passing through particularly spleen sinusoids.

### *2. Full Activation of Complement Cascade*

Some erythrocyte antibodies activate complement until C9 and makes holes in erythrocyte membrane. Natural antibodies of ABO system (IgM) and cold agglutinins (IgM) exemplify this action. Hemolysis is intravascular. Apart from IgM class antibodies, IgG1 and IgG3 class antibodies can also attach complement.

### *3. Cold Agglutination*

Cold antibodies whose thermal amplitude is high can agglutinate erythrocytes until 30-32°C degrees. This temperature which ensures agglutination is available in the surface capillary of end body parts like face, ears, and fingers which are exposed to cold. Thus, antibodies not only create vascular symptomatology of disease (acrocyanosis, even necrosis, livedo reticularis) but also attach complement components to erythrocyte surface [38]. When circulating blood returns to the centre at 37°C degrees, complement remains in the cellular surface although antibody is departed and thus agglutination is dissolved.

If antibody titer is too high, some cells can undergo hemolysis (intravascular hemolysis) after the completion of complement activation. Thus, hemoglobinuria and hemosiderinuria (at times of chronic phenomena) are observed. As mentioned above cells covered with C3b can be phagocyted after being caught by macrophages. This kind of macrophages is mainly found in liver and thus patients cannot benefit from splenectomy.

However, in most of the cells as a result of the inactivation of C3b, there remains only C3d on the cellular surface. Cells with Cd3 cannot be removed as macrophages do not have C3d receptors. Therefore, new complement activation cannot start in circulating erythrocytes covered with C3d when they encounter antibodies. That is why only young erythrocytes can undergo hemolysis. Because of that extreme reticuloytosis is not observed in cold agglutinin disease. On the other hand, C3d remaining on the circulating cells make direct Coombs test positive with the help of immune serum prepared against complement.

Donath-Landsteiner antibody, which is responsible for the hemolysis in paroxysmal cold hemoglobinuris, cannot agglutinate erythrocytes at low temperatures as they belong to IgG class. On the other hand, they adhere to erythrocytes the first components of complement at low temperatures. Intravascular hemolysis, which develops as a result of the completion of complement activation, takes place at 37°C. Therefore, Donald-Landsteiner antibody is also called “bisaphic antibody.”

# HEMOLYTIC TRANSFUSION REACTIONS

## Early Transfusion Reactions

American Association of Blood Banks (AABB) stated that any adverse effect on the patient during transfusion must be suspected to be transfusion reaction. This reaction should be evaluated if new symptoms appear or present symptoms become heavier on the blood transfusion recipients.

Transfusion reactions may occur at early or later periods and may be dependent on immune mechanisms and several other reasons [39].

Earlt transfusion reactions appear on 2% of all transfusions. Most frequent ones are mild, yet complications such as fluid load and hemolytic reactions bear the risk of mortality and morbidity. Most of these reactions derive from preventable human errors. Contamination risk of infections such as HIV and Hepatitis C are rapidly decreasing and it was stated that the pace of contamination plunged to one every 2 million transfusions.

## Hemolytic Transfusion Reactions due to Immune Mechanisms (Acute Hemolytic Transfusion Reactions)

Acute hemolytic transfusions are the most imminent side effects. The most widespread reason for this is false blood type transfusions due to easily preventable register errors. The manifestation could be in diverse ways such as sudden cardiovascular collapse leading to death, anemia as a result of hemolysis and adventitious asymptomatic events. Hemolytic reactions could be classified as intravascular and extravascular. Intravascular hemolysis occurs due to the precipitation of the whole cascade by the activation of the compliment and the destruction of erythrocite membrane by membrane attack complex. On the other side, ectravascular homolysis occurs by the phagocytosis of antibody covered erythrocides in *reticuloendothelial* system, spleen and other organs. The most common symptom of hemolytic reaction is shivering with fever. Tachypnea, respiratory disorder, cyanosis, pain in the infusion area, chest, back or waist, pain in abdomin, agitation, hyptension and shock may appear. Hemoglobinuria, anuria and oliguria may develop. Common bleeding may appear as the first symptom since other symptoms are repressed. Initial symptoms are dependent on the amount of the blood given. 5-20 ml a false blood type given to the patient may cause hemolytic reaction symptoms and mortality is bound to the amount. While mortality risk is 25% for 500-1000 ml transfusion, the rate increases to 44% for amounts over 1000ml. Agents starting hemolytic reactions are usually ABO izoaglutinines and sometimes are alloanti-cores against other antigens such as RH, Kell and Duffy. Fatal hemolytic reaction incidence is evaluated as 1 in every 1.000.000 transfusion. The distinctive diagnosis of hemolytic reactions includes effects of medicine, congenital hemolytic anemies, and acute hemolysis causing other conditions such as microangiopathic hemolysis. The diagnosis is confirmed by the examination of intravascular hemolysis, serum haptoglobin, *lactate* dehydrogenase (LHD) and indirect biliburine levels and and by the display of other serological anomality. The blood that caused reaction must be sent to the blood bank, samples pre and post transfusion must be examined in terms of hemolysis and the blood type test must be repeated, Coombs test must be given, blood samples must be cross checked and register errors must be questioned.

Immune complexes which occur due to erythrocite damage may harm renal tubuls and this leads to kidney function disorder, olyguria and anuria. In order to avoid this situation, shock must be prevented by liquid replacement and diuretics such as furosemide and mannitol must be used.

Tissue factor released from damaged erythrocite may initiate common diffuse intravascular coagulation (DIC). Coagulation tests like Protrombine time (PT), active partial tromboplastine time (APTT) and platelet amount must be examined in patients with hemolytic reaction.

## Non-Hemolytic Febrile Transfusion Reactions

Non-hemolytic febrile transfusions are the most frequent transfusion reactions. Initial symptoms are; increase in body temperature over 1°C and headache without being bound to any other reasons. Increase in temperature may go together with shivering. This consists of 43-74% of all transfusion reactions. These reactions are caused by donor leucocytes and antibodies against HLA antigens. Therefore, previous multi transfusion application and multiparous motherhood are accepted as risk factors. It is only possible to confirm febrile reaction diagnosis for increase in temperature by exclusion of other reasons such as hemolytic and septic reactions. Non-hemolytic reactions are observed in 15% of patients.

It is possible to prevent sensitization against platelet antigens by removing platelets in blood and in this way febril reaction incidence could be lowered. As cytokine released from bank blood cells may cause febrile reactions, platelets must be removed before preservation.

While paracetamol and meperidine could be used fort he cures of shivering along with temperature, antihistaminics are contradictive.

## Allergic Transfusion Reactions

An allergic reaction which begins with urticaria may progress to "wheezing" and anaphylaxis [40]. This occurs due to s formed against proteins in donor plasm. Antibodies against serum proteins, especially IgA is considered to be the main factor. Patients who had allergic reactions are under greater risk. It may be necessary to use washed erythrocite suspension. Oral and parenteral antihistaminics (difenhydramin 50 mg) could be given prophylactically or for treatment.

## Anaphylactic Transfusion Reactions

Symptoms of anaphylactic transfusion reactions are feeling bad, flushing of the skin, urticaria, larynx edema, and bronchospasm [41]. Severe hypotension, shock and heart arrest could occur. It is assumed that the reaction develops by unknown allergens or being dependent on anti IGA antibodies for patients who lack IgA. For patients prone to reactions, even amounts lower than 10 ml can lead to reactions. Transfusion must be terminated in case of any doubt.

## Transfusion-Related Acute Lung Infection (TRALI)

Transfusion-related acute lung infection causes non-cardiogenic lung edema [42]. However, due to insufficient knowledge on TRIALI and the difficulty of distinguishing the case from acute respiratory distress syndrome (ARDS), the number of cases notified remainv much below the actual number [43]. The manifestation consists of symptoms such as respiratory distress, cyanosis, coughing and symptoms of edema on both sides of the lung. Symptoms are sudden and severe, and most frequently appear in the first few hours following transfusion. Severity of the manifestation is dependent upon the level of hypoxia and causes morbidity significantly and is in third place in transfusion mortality. TRALI etyology and pathogenesis is the increase in capillary permeability and sequestration of platelets into lung tissue as a result of reaction of platelet antibodies formed in the blood of multiparous donors, with receptive platelets [44]. It was found that among the 70% of the cases at least one donor had granulocyte and HLA class antibodies [45]. In some cases, In some cases, HLA class II antibodies were found in donor plasm against the receiver's cells. Another hypothesis about the patogenesis is the capillary damage is considered to be bound to biologically active lipids which are formed by fragmentation of cells in the bak blood [46]. TRALI occurs by whole blood, erythrocide suspension, and fresh-frozen plasma transfusion [47]. Yet, it was stated in several publications that there exist TRALI cases that develop following reception of granulocyte, cryopresipitate and platelet suspension [48].

In hypoxia following transfusion and in lung graphic, TRALI must be evaluated from the point of infitrasyon not connected to heart failure and excessive liquid load [49]. Treatment begins with the termination of transfusion and continues as support treatment [50]. In order to eliminate respiratory distress, usually mechanical ventilation is necessary. TRALI cases are usually benign compared to ARDS cases and patients recover in a few days [51].

## Transfusion Reaction not Related to Nonimmune Mechanisms

These reactions are bound to mecahnical, chemical and bacteria contamination. Nonimmunologic reaction diagnosis is usually confirmed when post transfusion antibody search is negative.

Erythrocides may become hemolyzed due to excessive flow pace and pressure. Very high or very low temperature casuses thermal damage in erythrocides. Erythrocides may only be mixed with 0,0% sodium chloride. Apart from this, mixing erythrocides with hypo and hypertonic cristalloids, lactated ringer solution and with any other medicine damages them.

Massive transfusions lead to hypothermia, citrate toxidity, hemostasis disorder, potassium imbalance, acid-base imbalance and circulatory overload.

## Acute Bacterial Transfusion Reaction

Acute bacterial transfusion reactions occur due to contamination of blood by bacteria, infection of donor, using a technique other than aseptic during reception, improper preservation conditions, ignoring rules during transportation and exceeding the suggested 4 hour transfusion period. PLatelet suspensions preserved in room temperature have greater risk than other components. A recent study reveals that fatality due to bacteria contamination is one in 6 million erythrocide suspensions yet, the same rate is one in 200.000-300.000 in platelet suspension. The most significant symptoms are fever, shock, pain in any part of the body, and hemoglobinuria. Blood components must be carefully examined and products with gas formation, colour change, hemolysis in plasm and clot must certainly be avoided of use.

## Late Complications Related to Blood Transfusion

The need for transfusion has increased as the chronic disorders in the old population has recently been on the rise [52]. Nevertheless, blood donation is on the decline, and its cost is ever-increasing because of the new scan tests. The world has been acting in the direction of the motto "Blood saves lives." However, the risk of HIV and Hepatitis contaminated through transfusion has dramatically affected this trend. Although this shockwave has not been relieved yet, new disorders have started to be defined, which can be named such as Acute lung injury, immunomodulation related to transfusion, the increase in the risk of nosocomial infection, the increase of cancer recurrence and autoimmune disorders. All such factors have called the safety of blood and blood products transfusion into question and caused the review of transfusion practice.

Complications related to blood and blood products can be categorized into two as the early one and the late one. The late transfusion complications can be grouped into two as immunologic ones and the non immunologic ones. Late blood transfusion complications are delayed hemolytic transfusion reaction, transfusion related Graft-versus-Host Disroder (TR-GVHD), post-transfusion purpura, iron overload and immunomodulation due to transfusion.

## Delayed Hemolytic Transfusion Reactions

The ratio (1/500) one among about 500 erythrocytes is seen mostly in women. The reaction is low, and following the transfusion it is possible to encounter cases such as the drop in hematocrit, hemoglobinuria, jaundice and kidney function deficiencies [53]. Generally these cases are not fatal and they do not require any treatment. The antibodies can cause problems in the later transfusions. Therefore, the patient should be recorded and informed. The medical warning card should be given to the patient so that this situation will be taken into consideration in the transfusions to be enacted ahead.

## Transfusion Related Graft Versus Host Disease (TR-GVHD)

This is a rare incidence (with a frequency of 1/750.000 cellular blood product transfusion), however it is a fatal one [54]. It occurs when the immune system of the recipient is disrupted (allograft bone marrow transfusion, Hodgkin Disease, fetus with intrauterine transfusion), with a high similarity of HLA between the donor and the recipient (cases of being relatives) and transfusion of blood components with high amounts of T lymphocyte. Cell damage occurs when the T lymphocytes of the donor and the recipient's cells carrying Class I and Class II HLA antigens interact. The essential tissues are skin, thymus, gastrointestinal system, liver, spleen and bone marrow [55].

TR-GVHD might occur after the complete blood, erythrocyte suspension, platelet suspension and granulocyte suspension are delivered. Lymphocytes are fewer in the recently frozen plasma but this might be problematic for those afflicted with congenital immune deficiency. The frozen erythrocytes, cryoprecipitate, coagulation factors, albumin and IV immunoglobins with TR-GVHD have not been defined [56].

Clinical findings are at the onset after 1-2 weeks (4-30 days). These can be listed as the following: fever, maculopapular skin rashes, enterecolitis with diarrhea, hepatitis with increase in alkaline phosphates and bilirubins, as wel as hyperplasia and pancytopenia with decrease in all marrow elements. Lymphadenopathy and splenomegaly might be seen in the earlier periods in neonatals. Death occurs due to infection, amounting to more than 90 % of the cases.

The diagnosis is enabled through blood/blood component transfusion anamnesis, clinical findings and skin biopsy. The skin biopsy findings are not pathognomonic, they are rather supplementary. The display of donor lymphocyte permanency through cytogenetic and HLA analysis might prove beneficial but they do not yield exact results. The reason for this is that the donor lymphocytes have been reported to have been found in the recipient's blood within 1 week in adults, within 6-8 weeks in neonatals and within 2 years following intrauterine transfusion without an incidence of TR-GVHD. TR-GVDH does not have an effective treatment [57]. The Gama ray of the blood products with cells prevents TR-GVHD. Single does of 25 Gy erythrocyte prevents the multiplication of the lymphocytes without disrupting the functions of granulocyte and platelets. In cases where the donor has a kinship with the recipient, the blood products should be radiated through at least 25 Gy if blood component intrauterine is to be used, the immune system of the recipient is disrupted, the recipient has been exposed to allogenic bone marrow or peripheral root cell transplantation.

In recipients with Hodgkin Disease, neonatal blood transfusion, intense chemotherapy and radiotherapy, ones with bone marrow suppression (with absolute lymphocyte count less than 500 in mL) blood products containing radiated cell can be used. The reduction of leukocytes through filtration is a controversial issue.

## Transfusion Related Immunomodulation (TRIM)

A vast amount of antigen is loaded into the recipient through allogenic donor blood transfusion, which contains both high amounts of soluble and cellular foreign antigen [58]. This antigen load causes disruptions in the immunity. When the blood products are postponed, histamine, lipids, cytokines, cell membrane elements might dissolve.

Many active substances occur like the leukocyte of human antigen (HLA), Class I, etc. Most of them are derived from white blood cells (WBC) and they play a significant role in contributing to the formation of TRIM [59].

Potent proenflammatory cytokines like (RBC), IL-1, IL-6, IL-8, protein increasing bactericidal permeability and TNF-alpha occur in the stored erythrocytes, too. For this reason, it has been shown that neutrophile activation is triggered, IL-8, secretor phospholipid A2 is secreted and tendency to SIRS increases when stored erythrocytes are delivered. As the number of white blood cells in the erythrocyte suspension increases so does hemolysis. In addition, potassium comes out. Moreover, leukocyte apoptosis and toxic oxygen radicals increase. Arginase released from the stored erythrocytes is a significant intermediary agent substance in transfusion related immunosuppression.

After the finding which revealed in the early 1970's that renal allograft, rejection with allogenic blood transfusion decreased, it was further put forth in 1980's that tumor recurrence increased following the malign tumor resection. In the following years it was claimed that post-operative bacterial infection risk increased, activating cytonmegalovirus and HIV virus infections. All these findings show that allogenic blood transfusion causes TRIM.

The occurrence mechanism of TRIM has not been clarified entirely yet. It is considered that many biological mechanisms have an influence [60]. It has been shown in the animals used in experiments that soluble or cellular foreign antigen infusion cause immune suppression, anergia and clonal deletion. It is not clear yet whether specific allogenic blood products cause TRIM. Allogenic plasma, allogenic WBC and substances accumulating in the blood components during storage play roles in TRIM pathogenesis.

It has been set forth that the following combination of immunologic incidents causes TRIM pathogenesis [61, 62]:

a. The clonal deletion of cytotoxic T lymphocyte precursors and the change of T-cell repertoire.
b. Suppressor cell induction,
c. The suppression of NK cell activity,
d. The activation of cytokine production (IL2, IL4, IL1)
e. CD4+T cell decrease and decrease in the amount of CD4/CD8,
f. The existence of micro-chimerism between the recipient and the donor.

The immunity is suppressed, post-operation infections increase, wound healing decreases, viral infections are activated and cancer recurrence rises related to TRIM developing after allogenic transfusion whatever the reason is.

## Conclusion

The definition of ABO blood group antigens has been one of the most significant steps taken in the direction of safe transfusion. Anti-A or anti-B antibodies can cause intravascular hemolysis when ABO-incompatible erythrocytes are transfused. A and B antigens also are expressed on most tissue cells. For this reason, ABO compatibility is a significant consideration in hematopoietic stem cell transplantation, and solid organ transplantation.

## References

[1] Lewis, M., Anstee, D.J., Bird, G.W.G., Brodheim, E., Cartron, J.P., Contreras, M., et al. (1990) Blood group terminology 1990. The ISBT Working Party on Terminology for Red Cell Surface Antigens. *Vox Sang*, 58,152-69.

[2] Daniels, G.L., Fletcher, A., Garratty, G., Henry, S., Jørgensen, J., Judd, W.J., et al. (2004) Blood group terminology 2004: from the International Society of Blood Transfusion committee on terminology for red cell surface antigens. *Vox Sang*, 87, 304-16.

[3] Standards Committee of American Association of Blood Banks: Standards for Blood Banks and Transfusion Services (2003) 22nd ed. American Associations of Blood Banks, Bethesda.

[4] Roitt, I., Brostoff, J., Male, D.K., Immunology (2001) 6th ed. Mosby, London.

[5] Cartron, J.P., Colin, Y. (2001) Structural and functional diversity of blood group antigens. *Transfus Clin. Biol*, 8, 163-199.

[6] Brecher, M., ed. Technical Manual (2005) 15th ed., Bethesda, MD: American Association of Blood Banks.

[7] Daniels, G.L., Fletcher, A., Garratty, G., et al. (2004) Blood group terminology (2004): from the International Society of Blood Transfusion committee on terminology for red cell surface antigens. *Vox Sang*, 87, 304-316.

[8] Lögdberg, L., Reid, M.E., Lamont, R.E., Zelinski T. (2005) Human blood group genes 2004: chromosomal locations and cloning strategies. *Transfus Med. Rev*, 19, 45-57.

[9] Reid, M.E., Lomas-Francis, C. (2004) Blood Group Antigen FactsBook, 2nd ed. San Diego, Academic Press.

[10] Reid, M.E., Qyen, R., Marsh, W.L. (2000) Summary of the clinical significance of blood group alloantibodies. *Semin. Hematol*, 37, 197-216.

[11] Daniels, G., Poole, J., deSilva, M., Callaghan T, MacLennan S, Smith N. (2002) The clinical significance of blood group antibodies. *Transfus Med*, 12, 287-295.

[12] Reid, M.E., Lomas-Francis, C. (2007) Blood Group Antigens and Antibodies: A Guide to Clinical Relevance and Technical Tips, New York, Star Bright Books.

[13] Hillyer, C.D., et al (eds) (2006) Blood Banking and Transfusion Medicine: Basic Principles and Practices, 2d ed. Philadelphia, Churchill Livingstone.

[14] Hosoi, E. (2008) Biological and clinical aspects of ABO blood group system. *J. Med. Invest.,* 55:174-182.

[15] Nydegger, U.E., Tevaearai, H., Berdat, P., Rieben, R., Carrel, T., Mohacsi, P., Flegel, W. (2006) Histo-blood group antigens as allo- and auto-antigens. *Ann. N. Y. Acad. Sci.,* 1050:40-51.

[16] Smart, E., Armstrong, B. (2008) Blood group systems. *ISBT Sci. Series,* 3(2):68-92.

[17] Garratty, G., Dzik, W., Issitt, P.D., Lublin, D.M., Reid, M.E., Zelinski, T. (2000) Terminology for blood group antigens and genes – historical origins and guidelines in the new millennium. *Transfusion,* 40:477-489.

[18] Lögdberg, L., Reid, M.E., Miller, J.L. (2002) Cloning and genetic characterization of blood group carrier molecules and antigens. *Transfus Med. Rev*, 16, 1-10.

[19] Daniels, G. (2002) Human Blood Groups, 2nd ed. Blackwell Science, Oxford.

[20] Reid, M.E., Lomas-Francis, C. (2003) Blood Group Antigen Facts Book, 2nd ed. Academic, San Diego.

[21] Cartron, J.P., Colin, Y. (2001) Structural and functional diversity of blood group antigens. *Transfus Clin. Biol*, 8, 163-199.

[22] Reid, M.E., Mohandas, N. (2004) Red blood cell blood group antigens: Structure and function. *Semin. Hematol*, 41, 93-117.

[23] Brecher, M.E., Combs, M.R., Drew, M.J., et al. (2002) Technical Manual, 14th ed. American Association of Blood Banks, Bethesda.

[24] Daniels, G.L., Cartron, J.P., Fletcher, A., et al. (2003) International Society of Blood Transfusion Committee on terminology for red cell surface antigens: Vancouver report. *Vox Sang*, 84, 244-247.

[25] Avent, N.D., Reid, M.E. (2000) The Rh blood group system: a review. *Blood*, 95, 375-387.

[26] Tippett, P., Lomas-Francis, C., Wallace, M. (1996) The Rh antigen D: partial D antigens and associated low incidence antigens. *Vox Sang*, 70, 123-131.

[27] Westhoff, C.M. (2007) The structure and function of the Rh antigen complex. *Semin. Hematol*, 44, 42-50.

[28] Avent, N.D., Madgett, T.E., Lee, Z.E., Head, D.J., Maddocks, D.G., Skinner, L.H. (2006) Molecular biology of Rh proteins and relevance to molecular medicine. *Expert Rev. Mol. Med.,* 8(13):1-20.

[29] Montano, R.F., Penichet, M.L., Blackall, D.P., Morrison, S.L., Chintalacharuvu, K.R. (2009) Recombinant polymeric IgG anti-Rh: a novel strategy for development of direct agglutinating reagents. *J. Immunol. Methods*, 340, 1-10.

[30] Marsh, W.L., Redman, C.M. (1990) The Kell blood group system: a review. *Transfusion*, 30, 158-167.

[31] Lee, S., Russo, D., Redman, C.M. (2000) The Kell blood group system: Kell and XK membrane proteins. *Semin. Hematol*, 37, 113-121.

[32] Lee, S. (1997) Molecular basis of Kell blood group phenotypes. *Vox Sang*, 73, 1-11.

[33] Reid, M.E., Mohandas, N. (2004) Red blood cell blood group antigens: structure and function. *Semin. Hematol*, 41, 93-117.

[34] Mohandas, N., Narla, A. (2005) Blood group antigens in health and disease. Curr. Opin. Hematol, 12, 135-40.

[35] Learoyd, P., Knight, R. (2002) Introduction to Blood Transfusion Science and Blood Bank Practice.

[36] Zeng, J.Q., Deng, Z.H., Yang, B.C., Liang, Y.L., Su, Y.Q., Li da, C., Yu, Q. (2009) Polymorphic analysis of the Lutheran blood group system in Chinese. *Ann. Clin. Lab. Sci*, 39, 38-42.

[37] Brand, A. (2002) Immunological aspects of blood transfusions. *Transplant Immunol*, 10, 183-190.

[38] Petz, L.D., Garratty, G. (2003) Acquired Immune Hemolytic Anemias, 2nd ed. Churchill Livingstone, New York.

[39] Ambrusso, D.R. (2003) Hemolytic transfusion reactions. In Hillyer CD, Silberstein LE, Ness PM, eds. Blood Banking and Transfusion Medicine. Basic Principles and Practice. New York: Chuchill Livingstone, pp 391-4.

[40] Domen, R.E., Hoeltge, G.A. (2003) Allergic transfusion reactions: an evaluation of 273 consecutive reactions. *Arch Pathol. Lab. Med*, 127, 316-320.

[41] Stack, E., Pomper, G.J. (2002) Febrile, allergic, and nonimmune transfusion reactions. In: Simon TL, Dzik WH, Snyder EL, et al ed. Rossi's Principles of Transfusion Medicine, Philadelphia: Lippincott Williams and Wilkins, 831.

[42] Marik, P.E. (2009) The hazards of blood transfusion. *Br. J. Hosp. Med. (Lond)*, 70, 12-15.

[43] Silliman, C.C., Boshkov, L.K., Mehdizadehkashi, Z., Elzi, D.J., Dickey, W.O., Podlosky, L., Clarke, G., Ambruso, D.R. (2003) Transfusion-related acute lung injury: epidemiology and a prospective analysis of etiologic factors. *Blood*, 101, 454- 462.

[44] Kopko, P.M., Paglieroni, T.G., Popovsky, M.A., Muto, K.N., MacKenzie, M.R., Holland, P.V. (2003) TRALI: correlation of antigen-antibody and monocyte activation in donor-recipient pairs. *Transfusion*, 43, 177-84.

[45] Kopko, P.M., Popovsky, M.A., MacKenzie, M.R., Paglieroni TG, Muto KN, Holland PV. (2001) HLA class II antibodies in transfusion-related acute lung injury. Transfusion, 41(10):1244-1248.

[46] Sheppard, C.A. et al. (2007) Transfusion-related acute lung injury. *Hematol. Oncol. Clin. North Am*, 21, 163-176.

[47] Clark, C.T. (2009) Transfusion-related acute lung injury: clinical features and diagnostic dilemmas. *J Infus Nurs*, 32, 132-136.

[48] Kopko, P.M., Marshall, C.S., MacKenzie, M.R., Holland PV, Popovsky MA. (2002) Transfusion-related acute lung injury: report of a clinical look-back investigation. *JAMA*, 287, 1968-1971.

[49] Popovsky, M.A. (2000) Transfusion-related acute lung injury. *Curr. Opin. Hematol*, 7, 402-407.

[50] Silliman, C.C., Boskhov, L.K., Mehdizadehkashi, Z., et al. (2003) Transfusion-related acute lung injury: epidemiology and a prospective analysis of etiologic factors. *Blood*, 101, 454-462.

[51] Looney, M.R., Gropper, M.A., Mathay, M.A. (2004) Transfusion-related acute lung injury: a review. *Chest*, 26, 249-258.

[52] Miller, R.D. (2005) Transfusion Therapy. In: Miller's Anesthesia. Ed: Miller RD. Sixth Ed.Elsevier, Philadelphia. 1799-1830.

[53] Simmons, E.D. (2002) Transfusion therapy. In: Current Critical Care Diagnosis and Treatment. Eds. Bongart FS, Sue DY. Second Ed., Lange, 78-95.

[54] Linden, J.V., Wagner, K., Voytovich, A.E., Sheehan, J. (2000) Transfusion errors in New York State: an analysis of 10 years' experience. *Transfusion*, 40, 1207-1213.

[55] Ahrens, N., Pruss, A., Kahne, A., Kiesewetter, H., Salama, A. (2007) *Transfusion*, 47, 813-816.

[56] Carey, P.M., Sacher, R.A. (2002) Transfusion-associated graft versus host disease. In: Simon TL, Dzik WH, Snyder EL, et al ed. Rossi's Principles of Transfusion Medicine, Philadelphia: Lippincott Williams and Wilkins, 852.

[57] Webb, I.J., Anderson, K.C. (2001) Transfusion-associated graft vs. host disease. In: Popovsky MA, ed. Transfusion Reactions, Bethesda, MD: AABB Pres, 171.

[58] Blajchman, M.A. (2002) Immunomodulation and blood transfusion. *Am. J. Ther*, 9, 389-395.

[59] Blajchman, M.A., Dzik, S., Vamvakas, E.C., Sweeney, J., Synder, E.L. (2001) Clinical and molecular basis of transfusion-induced immunomodulation: summary of the proceedings of a state-of-the-art conference. *Transfus Med. Rev*, 15, 108.

[60] Rouger, P. (2004) Transfusion induced immunomodulation: myth or reality? *Transfus Clin. Biol*, 11, 115-116.

[61] Bluth, M.H., Reid, M.E., Manny, N. (2007) Chimerism in the immunohematology laboratory in the molecular biology area. *Transfus. Med. Rev.*, 21(2):134-146.

[62] Vamvakas, E.C., Blajchman, M.A. (2007) Transfusion-related immunomodulation (TRIM): An update. *Blood Rev.*, 21(6):327-48.

# INDEX

## B

## C

## D



## E

## F



## G

## H

## I

## K



## L

## M

## N



## O

## P

## R

## S

# T

## U

## V



## W



## X



## Y



## Z